# THE POISONER'S HANDBOOK

# THE POISONER'S HANDBOOK

## MURDER AND THE BIRTH OF FORENSIC MEDICINE IN JAZZ AGE NEW YORK

## DEBORAH BLUM

**THORNDIKE PRESS**
*A part of Gale, Cengage Learning*

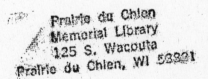
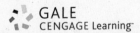
GALE
CENGAGE Learning

Detroit • New York • San Francisco • New Haven, Conn • Waterville, Maine • London

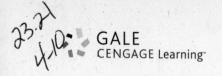

**GALE**
CENGAGE Learning™

**LIBRARY OF CONGRESS CATALOGING-IN-PUBLICATION DATA**

Blum, Deborah, 1954–
    The poisoner's handbook : murder and the birth of forensic medicine in jazz age New York / by Deborah Blum. — Large print ed.
        p. cm.
    Includes bibliographical references.
    ISBN-13: 978-1-4104-2512-6 (hardcover : alk. paper)
    ISBN-10: 1-4104-2512-6 (hardcover : alk. paper)
    1. Poisoning—New York (State)—History. 2. Forensic toxicology—New York (State)—History. 3. Forensic science—New York (State)—History. 4. Large type books. I. Title.
    HV6555.U52N373 2010b
    614'.1309747109041—dc22                                    2009053951

Published in 2010 by arrangement with The Penguin Press, a member of Penguin Group (USA) Inc.

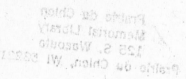

Printed in the United States of America
1 2 3 4 5 6 7 14 13 12 11 10

*To the Haugen family — Dave, Helen, Peter (always), Treaka — and in loving memory of Pamela.*

# CONTENTS

# PROLOGUE:
## THE POISON GAME

Until the early nineteenth century few tools existed to detect a toxic substance in a corpse. Sometimes investigators deduced poison from the violent sickness that preceded death, or built a case by feeding animals a victim's last meal, but more often than not poisoners walked free. As a result murder by poison flourished. It became so common in eliminating perceived difficulties, such as a wealthy parent who stayed alive too long, that the French nicknamed the metallic element arsenic *poudre de succession,* the inheritance powder.

The chemical revolution of the 1800s changed the relative ease of such killings. Scientists learned to isolate and identify the basic elements and the chemical compounds that define life on Earth, gradually building a catalog, *The Periodic Table of the Elements.* In 1804, the elements palladium, cerium, iridium, osmium, and rhodium were discov-

9

ered; potassium and sodium were isolated in 1807; barium, calcium, magnesium, and strontium in 1808; chlorine in 1810. Once researchers understood individual elements they went on to study them in combination, examining how elements bonded to create exotic compounds and familiar substances, such as the sodium-chlorine combination that creates basic table salt (NaCl).

The pioneering scientists who worked in elemental chemistry weren't thinking about poisons in particular. But others were. In 1814, in the midst of this blaze of discovery, the Spanish chemist Mathieu Orfila published a treatise on poisons and their detection, the first book of its kind. Orfila suspected that metallic poisons like arsenic might be the easiest to detect in the body's tissues and pushed his research in that direction. By the late 1830s the first test for isolating arsenic had been developed. Within a decade more reliable tests had been devised and were being used successfully in criminal prosecutions.

But the very science that made it possible to identify the old poisons, like arsenic, also made available a lethal array of new ones. Morphine was isolated in 1804, the same year that palladium was discovered. In 1819 strychnine was extracted from the seeds of the Asian vomit button tree (*Strychnos nux vomica*). The lethal compound coniine was isolated from hemlock the same year. Chemists neatly extracted nicotine from tobacco leaves in 1828. Aconitine — described by one toxicologist as "in its pure state, perhaps the most potent poison known" — was found in the beautifully flowering monkshood plant in 1832.

And although researchers had learned to isolate these alkaloids — organic (carbon-based) compounds with some nitrogen mixed in — they had no idea how to find such poisons in human tissue. Orfila himself, conducting one failed attempt after another, worried that it was an impossible task. One exasperated French prosecutor, during a mid-nineteenth-century trial involving a morphine murder, exclaimed: "Henceforth let us tell would-be poisoners; do not use metallic poisons for they leave traces. Use plant poisons . . . Fear nothing; your crime will go unpunished. There is no corpus delecti [physical evidence] for it cannot be found."

So began a deadly cat and mouse game — scientists and poisoners as intellectual adversaries. A gun may be fired in a flash of anger, a rock carelessly hurled, a shovel swung in sudden fury, but a homicidal poisoning requires a calculating intelligence. Unsurprisingly, then, when metallic poisons, such as arsenic, became detectable in bodies, informed killers turned away from them. A survey of poison prosecutions in Britain found that, by the mid-nineteenth century, arsenic killings were decreasing. The trickier plant alkaloids were by then more popular among murderers.

In response, scientists increased their efforts to capture alkaloids in human tissue. Finally, in 1860, a reclusive and single-minded French chemist, Jean Servais Stas, figured out how to isolate nicotine, an alkaloid of the tobacco plant, from a corpse. Other plant poisons soon became more accessible and chemists were able to offer new assistance to criminal investigations. The field of toxicology was becoming something to be reckoned with, especially in Europe.

The knowledge, and the scientific determination, spread across the Atlantic to the United States. The 1896 book *Medical Jurisprudence, Forensic Medicine and Toxicology*, cowritten by a New York research chemist and a law professor, documented the still-fierce competition between scientists and killers. In one remarkable case in New York, a physician had killed his wife with morphine and then put belladonna drops into her eyes to counter the telltale contraction of her pupils. He was convicted only after Columbia University chemist Rudolph Witthaus, one of the authors of the 1896 text, demonstrated the process to the jury by killing a cat in the courtroom using the same gruesome technique. There was as much showmanship as science, Witthaus admitted; toxicology remained a primitive field of research filled with "questions still unanswerable."

In the early twentieth century industrial innovation flooded the United States with a wealth of modern poisons, creating new opportunities for the clever poisoner and new challenges for the country's early forensic detectives. Morphine went into teething medicines for infants; opium into routinely prescribed sedatives; arsenic was an ingredient in everything from pesticides to cosmetics. Mercury, cyanide, strychnine, chloral hydrate, chloroform, sulfates of iron, sugar of lead, carbolic acid, and more, the products of the new chemistry stocked the shelves of doctors' offices, businesses, homes, pharmacies, and grocery stores. During the Great War poison was established as a weapon of warfare, earning World War I the name "The Chemist's War." And with the onset of Prohibition a new Chemist's War raged between bootleggers and government chemists working to make moonshine a lethal concoction. In New York's smoky jazz clubs, each round of cocktails became a game of Russian roulette.

There was no way for the barely invented science of toxicology to keep up with the deluge. Though a few dogged researchers were putting out manuals and compiling textbooks on the subject, too many novel compounds had yet to be analyzed and most doctors had little or no training in the subject.

In 1918, however, New York City made a radical reform that would revolutionize the poison game and launch toxicology into front-page status. Propelled by a series of scandals involving corrupt coroners and unsolved murders, the city hired its first trained medical examiner, a charismatic pathologist by the name of Charles Norris. Once in office, Norris swiftly hired an exceptionally driven and talented chemist named Alexander Gettler and persuaded him to found and direct the city's first toxicology laboratory.

Together Norris and Gettler elevated

forensic chemistry in this country to a formidable science. Trailblazing scientific detectives, they earned a respected place in the courtroom, crusaded against compounds dangerous to public health, and stopped a great many Jazz Age poisoners in their tracks. As they determinedly countered the obstacles faced in each new case they developed innovative laboratory methods for teasing toxins from human tissue. Their scientific contribution became a legacy for future generations.

But this story begins before Charles Norris or Alexander Gettler took office, before forensic toxicology was considered a fully legitimate science. It begins in the gray of a frozen January in the city, when an unlikely serial killer decided to make his move in the poison game.

# ONE:
## CHLOROFORM
## $(CHCl_3)$
### 1915

It would, of course, be in the cursed winter of 1915 — when ice storms had glassed over the city, when Typhoid Mary had come sneaking back, when the Manhattan coroner was discovered to be skunk-drunk at crime scenes — that the loony little porter would confess to eight poison murders.

At first the confession seemed just more of the general craziness spiking across the city. New York was mired in winter, horse-drawn carriages careening through snow-drifted Broadway, trolleys stuck in place from the Bronx to Coney Island as the weight of ice dragged down the lines. The streets commissioner had hired fifteen thousand "snow fighters," as he called them, to dig out the roadways. Even as the fighters shoveled and chopped, new snow dropped, new sleet kept falling, laying down yet another treacherous layer.

During those same days of darkening skies

and frozen streets, public authorities were desperately trying to stop a sudden outbreak of typhoid fever. The city's most notorious carrier, Typhoid Mary Mallon, had violated the conditions of her release from a sanitarium and gone to work as a cook at a local hospital. Twenty-five people were sick and two dead before they managed to hunt her down and take her — screaming and cursing them for persecution — back into custody.

The city's coroner had been no help in that investigation, if indeed he ever was.

Instead, Patrick Riordan was trying to fast-talk himself out of charges that he showed up for work sodden drunk. Or as one angry witness put it, he stumbled into a death scene with "a glassy eye and smirky face" to sneer at bodies. That indictment followed an accident on the Ninth Avenue Elevated, the crowded commuter line run by the private Interborough Rapid Transit Company.

The collision had occurred several weeks earlier, in the last days of December. Newspapers described it like a scene from a circle of hell — brakes failed on a local, metal and flame exploded as it went slamming into the back of an express waiting at the Eighth

Avenue and 116th Street station. The impact had pushed the wooden cars upward into a blazing pyramid. Flying sparks then set the platform on fire. Passengers, dazed and bloody, fled to the street, stumbling down the rickety stairs from the seventy-five-foot-high track, crowds gathering in the fire-lit dark to catch them if they fell. Two train workers died in the crash. Dozens more workers and passengers went to the hospital seeking treatment for burns, lacerations, and shock.

The papers also offered a memorable image of the coroner that night. Eight hours after the accident, as the hands of the clock were just slipping past two a.m., Riordan finally ambled into the police station where the bodies lay. An assistant was holding him upright, officers reported, and he was a big enough man that his weight pulled both of them sideways. Riordan looked down at the dead men. When told their names — Joseph Collins, 52, Gottlieb Minnick, 27 — he snapped, slurring the words but saying clearly enough: "It's a shame that two such names should pull us out on a night like this." All this according to the notes of journalists covering the accident, who helped trigger a formal investigation of Riordan's work.

Naturally it would be then, in January 1915, in the month of the drunken coroner, of snow fighters in the streets and cholera in the sick wards, that a self-proclaimed serial killer would walk into the district attorney's office, offering up his impossible tale of poison and murder.

Frederic Mors was a small man, short, thin, nervous. He had narrow blue eyes, slightly shaggy dark hair, and a beard dusted with cigarette ash. He smoked constantly, those aromatic Egyptian cigarettes, and he paced, paced, paced as he told his story. He was a recent immigrant from Vienna, and his English was slow, stumbling enough, that the police brought in an interpreter. "Oh, I wish I spoke English better," he exclaimed during the initial police interview, but the officers were able to piece together the story anyway.

He'd come over from Austria in early 1914, wanting to work in medicine. He'd found a job as an orderly at the German Odd Fellows home in Yonkers. The home, a refuge for 250 foundlings and one hundred elderly pensioners, paid only a little — $18 a month plus room and board — but allowed Mors to practice his medical interests. He was soon "made practically a nurse because the men over me realized that I knew something about nursing and was better educated than most orderlies." Shortly later, he said, the superintendent asked him to take on another job, to help with the "removal" of some of the sickliest, and costliest, residents.

In the interview room, Mors shrugged, lit another cigarette, and continued. The superintendent was a bully, he'd realized, and it was best to do what the man wanted. But this assignment, he explained carefully, didn't particularly bother him. "It was really a kind-hearted thing to do. They were all in great pain that could not be relieved. There was no chance for them. Also they were not pleasant physically or mentally to themselves or anyone else." The only challenge was deciding how to carry out the assignment. After reviewing the possibilities, he decided that poison was the obvious answer. In a place where people were old and unwell, it would be easy enough to make it look as if their time had simply come.

The home's nursing dispensary held a witch's closet of poisons, watched over by one of the young orphans, earning her keep. There were bottles filled with sugar of lead, those silvery crystals used to treat skin rashes; painkillers such as codeine, mor-

21

phine, and powdered opium; atropine, an extract from the nightshade plant, for speeding up a slowing heart; sweet-scented chloroform for anesthesia; white, powdery arsenic, for curing everything from syphilis to psoriasis; strychnine for energy tonics; and mercury for infections. The only question was which would best suit his purpose.

Mors first tried arsenic, but the elderly man selected for the experiment did not die in an orderly fashion. He was messily sick, then developed a kind of creeping paralysis, living on for several miserable days. Mors found himself on constant, exhausting nursing duty. It was horrible, he said, both for the victim and for himself. They buried the man — whatever his name was, he didn't remember — with great relief.

He went back to the dispensary. It was, maybe, the smell that decided him, that sweet chemical sting in the air, that sugary, seductive promise. He smiled at the detectives and told them why he'd been so pleased with his next choice: "When you give an old person chloroform, it's like putting a child to sleep."

There wasn't a cop in the room who thought of chloroform in terms of a lullaby.

Their experience was otherwise. They

knew it purely as a poison, one used by criminals, especially by thieves, who found it useful in robbing occupied homes. Since the turn of the twentieth century, this practice had been increasingly popular. Robbers would knock on an apartment door, force a chloroform-soaked rag over the face of whoever answered, and take what they wanted while their victim remained unconscious. "Burglar uses Chloroform: Attacks a Woman in a Flat, Robs Her and Cuts off her Hair," read one *New York Times* headline in March 1900. Beautiful hair for wigs was as valuable as some jewelry, the newspaper pointed out. And there were the burglars who "put an entire family under anesthetic" in 1907 before emptying their house; the train robbers who drugged a Pullman car full of passengers and emptied pockets and purses; the party host who put chloroform into his guests' drinks, then went through their wallets and disappeared with $3,000; and the robbers who chloroformed an attorney on a busy Manhattan street in 1910, yanked off his heavy gold and diamond ring, and disappeared into the crowd. Occasionally chloroform played a role in real tragedy; a Long Island father, in 1911, killed his son and two daughters with chloroform and then, leaving a suicide note, walked away into the gray Atlantic.

Mors liked chloroform for its efficiency. He'd used it to kill seven more residents with no problem at all. It was a wonderful poison, really, he said, perhaps a little cloying in its oversweet smell — but perfectly, reliably lethal.

The story went that the doctor who pioneered chloroform as an anesthetic had recognized its potential after it knocked him out cold. James Young Simpson, an Edinburgh physician, had been searching for something better than ether to relieve pain during surgery and childbirth. Ether could be frustratingly slow to act. Also it smelled awful, irritated the lungs, and was prone to ignite, which posed a definite risk at a time when surgeons often worked by candlelight.

Simpson and his two lab assistants decided to experiment on themselves until they found something that worked. They had already tried and dismissed compounds including acetone and benzene when, on the evening of November 4, 1847, they poured out tumblers of chloroform and dipped their faces into the vapor rising from the glass. Within two minutes all three were lying unconscious under the table, "in a trice under the mahogany," as Simpson later wrote. They awoke perhaps half an hour later, light-headed and dizzy but cheerfully unharmed. "This will change the world," he thought.

For the next five decades chloroform gained steadily in popularity. Every drugstore stocked it; most doctors, barring a few wary holdouts, prescribed it in abundance. It was mixed into cough syrups and liniments; it was dispensed as a sedative, a sleep aid, a painkiller, a treatment for alcoholic DTs, for hiccupping, seasickness, colic, vomiting, and diarrhea. No one was exactly sure how it worked, just that it appeared to slow the body down and sedate the brain, sliding a patient into a much-desired stupor.

The more physicians used chloroform, though, the more they realized that it was a capricious kind of anesthesia. There were reports of patients who inexplicably, unexpectedly died on the operating table before the surgeon even lifted his knife. An invalid would slide away into chloroform-induced unconsciousness and just keep sliding. The breathing would sputter to bare gasps; the heartbeats would decrease in an ever-slowing rhythm. Alarmed doctors began tallying the deaths. On average, it seemed, chloroform anesthesia killed at least one in every three thousand patients.

And no one knew how to fix that because no one was sure why it happened.

Chloroform was a simple enough compound, an uncomplicated arrangement of carbon, hydrogen, and chlorine. Yet somehow that tidy mixture formed a chemical loose cannon, killing without warning or apparent reason. Doctors weren't really even sure what a safe dose was. One patient died after receiving one-third of an ounce; another man, a known chloroform addict, succumbed only after going through a quart of the drug. Chloroform, not surprisingly, was riskiest for children, the elderly, and alcoholics, but it also, unpredictably, killed healthy adults.

At the turn of the twentieth century, the British Medical Association called chloroform the most dangerous anesthetic known, and the American Medical Association urged that hospitals stop using it entirely. But it would be several more decades before chloroform disappeared from the pharmacy shelves. At the time Frederic Mors lifted the bottle off the dispensary shelf, chloroform was still widely used, still known for being miraculous rather than murderous.

The police detectives in their dark wool suits became a familiar sight at the Odd Fellows Home, thumping down the wooden halls, opening closets, looking under beds, asking questions, checking out Mors's story. The more investigators looked and asked, the more they suspected the crazy little man might be telling the truth.

They found, for instance, a German poison manual hidden in the back of his closet. They gathered witnesses who confirmed some of his story, starting with the embalmer who worked at the funeral chapel serving the Odd Fellows home. Mors had told police that he'd put too much chloroform on the rag used to kill one elderly man. The caustic liquid left raw red marks around the man's mouth. The embalmer alarmed him by asking about the marks of injury. From then on, according to Mors's confession, he'd spread Vaseline around the patients' mouths before applying chloroform.

The embalmer promptly corroborated Mors's statement. He remembered being startled by that uneven red scoring of the skin. He'd seen chloroform burns on the faces of patients who'd died during surgery. Mors had told him a cloth used to tie the man's mouth shut after death had rubbed the face raw. That had puzzled the embalmer. The home had never done that before. The marks didn't really seem to match with a cloth burn. But after all, it was just another old man dead. And the next body showed no such signs of damage, so he'd let it go.

That led to another witness — an orderly who'd seen Mors rubbing Vaseline over an old man's face two hours before the patient was found dead. Mors had explained to him that the Vaseline would make it easier for the undertaker to shave the corpse. The orderly had been surprised — after all, the man was still breathing. Following that awkward encounter, Mors told the police, he'd switched to another method, pushing chloroform-soaked cotton wool into the noses of his chosen victims. When they searched Mors's room, officers found cotton and tweezers in the pocket of one of his coats.

The embalmer hadn't liked Mors. He found him competent but cold, "indifferent to the suffering and deaths of those in the home." The elderly residents hadn't liked him either. He had a reputation for threatening inmates who complained too much, who insisted on extra attention. The fourteen-year-old girl in charge of the medical dispensary told the police that Mors had commented to her about the uselessness of the residents, adding that it "would be a good thing" to get rid of a few of them. "If you don't stop making so much trouble, I'll send you to where there is more heat than you want," he had snapped at one ninety-one-year-old man.

The elderly residents at the home told police they believed Mors had methodically been removing those who annoyed him. They recalled him warning one woman who kept ringing her bell, requesting assistance, that she would be sorry if she summoned him again. She'd continued calling him. The next day she was dead.

But another orderly told police that he believed Mors had followed orders. Once the orderly had been summoned to help remove a dead patient from a room. When he reached the man's quarters, Mors and Superintendent Adam Banger were standing by the bed together, talking. There was a corpse in the bed, and the room had a sharp, sweet chemical sting to it. "What is it?" he remembered asking, choking slightly. In answer, Mors went to the window and threw it open. The superintendent lit a cigar, filling the air with the acrid burn of tobacco, erasing all trace of anything else.

The district attorney agreed that such interviews were suggestive. But from where he stood, they weren't proof. Now that Mors was in jail and the superintendent was locked up as a hostile and uncooperative witness, the mood at the Odd Fellows home had reached a predictable level of hysteria. Some of these statements were undoubtedly true, but others might be mere dramatics. To prove that these elderly residents had been poisoned, they needed some solid evidence.

No one, not even those who disliked him, claimed to have witnessed Mors killing a patient with chloroform. Rumors, suspicions, and anecdotes, a confession by a suspect who might just be crazy, weren't enough to charge a man with murder.

"Why did you shift from arsenic to chloroform?" the sheriff asked Mors.

"I did it because patients had become more troublesome after they had been given arsenic than before," Mors answered, during a hearing. "No person was ever killed unless he was going to die. I did it to end their suffering."

Investigators had thought at first that they could build their case on the arsenic murder. Arsenic is a tough, durable, metallic element. Traces of it could be found in corpses years after death. Their first plan was to dig up Mors's arsenic victim from the Bronx cemetery and run tests on whatever remained. But to their dismay, they discovered that the home was in the habit of dosing patients with an arsenic tonic, meaning that even if they did find the poison in tissue, it wouldn't necessarily provide evidence of murder.

As for chloroform, the coroner had sadly assured them all that there was no way, no way at all, to find evidence of it in a corpse. An autopsy, he said, was therefore a complete waste of time: "We might do this in some cases, but Mors has said that he chloroformed the persons he killed in Westchester, and the fact that a person has been chloroformed cannot be proven by an autopsy.

"Therefore we can establish nothing by exhuming the bodies. Mors may have given each of his victims a quart of chloroform but we couldn't prove it by an autopsy."

The worst-case example concerning the failure of an autopsy after a chloroform death came out of New York City's criminal justice history. It was the case of Texas multimillionaire William Rice, who might — or might not — have been killed with chloroform as he lay sleeping in his Manhattan apartment.

Rice died in the fall of 1900. The motive for his possible murder began with his decision, some years earlier, to found an educational institute in Houston. His fortune would eventually endow Rice University. But family members considered that his plans meant throwing their inheritance away. In fact, his wife, who died a few years before him, secretly made a will leaving her share of the estate to her relatives. As Texas was a community property state, her relatives then demanded half of Rice's own money.

Rice was eighty-four years old, an ailing and cantankerous recluse, burrowed into luxurious retirement. But he wanted to be remembered, he wanted his millions to endow his educational dream, and he had no intention of further subsidizing his wife's grasping relatives. Through his lawyers, he stated that he hadn't been a resident of Texas for years — he lived in New York, which was not a community property state. And his greedy relatives by marriage? Well, they could whistle for his money.

His wife's family, equally determined, countered by hiring a New York lawyer named Albert Patrick, who had a reputation for playing dirty. With his clients living halfway across the country, Patrick decided to siphon off some of Rice's money for himself. He developed an alliance with Rice's valet, Charles Jones, and they collaborated on a forged will that divided the old man's assets among the eager heirs, Jones, and of course, the attorney himself. The schemers then collaborated on getting rid of Rice.

Or so Jones claimed, once he was in jail, charged with chloroforming the old man at Patrick's bidding. The valet said he'd first tried mercury pills as a poison, but Rice seemed to thrive on them. So hearing that chloroform rapidly dissipated and left no evidence behind, he "borrowed" some from his brother, whose doctor had prescribed it as a sleep aid. According to his confession, Jones then put a chloroform-soaked sponge over his sleeping employer's face, anchored it with a heavy towel, and waited. Rice had died without a struggle, he claimed, and he burned the sponge and other equipment. Patrick arranged to have the body rushed to a crematorium.

From that point on, apparently, everything went wrong for the conspirators. The undertaker embalmed the body instead of incinerating it. The bank challenged the forged will that Patrick had provided and contacted the police. The suspicious coroner demanded an autopsy. The city decided to prosecute. Police had the faked documents, and a very dead millionaire. They then got Jones's confession. It seemed an easy path to conviction. They charged both Patrick and Jones with murder. As for Rice's body, city attorneys sent it to medical experts for what they expected to be a simple analysis.

But the Rice case proved cursed to all associated with it. Rumors spread that the valet had blamed Patrick in order to save himself, that he was unstable, seeing plots where there were none. The will was plainly forged, but many began to wonder whether Jones had built an attention-grabbing fantasy around Rice's natural death. When questioned, the valet became hysterical and staged a hunger strike in his jail cell, spicing up all those rumors of his mental instability.

Meanwhile the autopsy result turned out to be a catalog of contradictions. The body had started to rot. The doctors couldn't agree on how decomposition affected chloroform chemistry in the body. They couldn't agree on how embalming had changed the chemistry either. By the time the trial was over, more than $30,000 had been spent on experts who agreed on, well, nothing.

The autopsy, for instance, had found fluid in Rice's lungs. The defense called in one of the late President McKinley's doctors to assure jurors that chloroform was not a noxious, irritating substance that caused fluid to form in the lungs. The physician, while on the witness stand, pulled a small bottle of chloroform out of his pocket, held it under his tongue and his eyes, and declared that he hadn't felt a thing. The old man, he said, had died of pneumonia — it wasn't surprising that his lungs contained fluid. The physician was countered by a pathologist from Cornell who insisted that chloroform was strongly irritating and could rapidly cause the lungs to swell and fill. He blamed the poison, and the poison only, for Rice's congested lungs.

The next witness contradicted the Cornell pathologist, and so it continued until the jury simply dismissed the medical evidence, voting for conviction based on the valet's testimony and the forged documents. Jones was sentenced to life in prison, and Patrick was sentenced to death and sent to Sing Sing prison in 1902. But the convictions remained tainted by uncertainty. New York executions usually ticked along, Swiss-clock efficient, but Patrick's date with the electric chair kept getting pushed back. After four years the governor commuted his sentence to life, citing the unholy mess of medical arguments.

And in 1912 Patrick was pardoned, based largely on new statements from medical experts, saying that the autopsy evidence was inconclusive about the poison in question. "Doctors Say Chloroform Didn't Kill Rice," the New York papers wrote. All these years later, no one was sure if New York had wrongly convicted an innocent man or let a murderer go free.

That was the position they seemed to be in with Frederic Mors. They had no way to prove he was a murderer, and no way to be sure he wasn't. The Bronx district attorney decided that he had only one other avenue to pursue. If their self-confessed murderer really was crazy, if they could get a good alienist to diagnose him, they might not need the chloroform evidence. They could just have him safely put away. The DA decided to send the strange little suspect to Bellevue Hospital, home to the best psychopathic ward in the city, and possibly the entire country.

Like all other buildings in New York, Bellevue and Allied Hospitals wore a slick coat of ice that February, gleaming over the brick and stone, adding slippery polish to the wrought-iron gates and curved staircases, a cold winter sheen to the sedately styled Victorian buildings.

The Bellevue complex spread over four city blocks along the East River, built on land that had once nourished a farm called Belle Vue, for its beautiful prospect on the river. The first hospital building had been constructed there in 1811; only eight years later Bellevue became the first U.S. hospital to formally require a qualified physician to pronounce a death (after a desperately ill man had been discovered among the corpses stacked on the morgue wagon). Its ambulance system had started in 1869; its children's clinic (the first in the nation) in 1874; its chest clinic, to combat tuberculosis, in 1903. It was from the start a public hospital — in the winter of 1915, nearly a thousand people were treated at Bellevue every day. "It gathers the dead and dying from river and streets and is kept busy night and day with the misery of the living," wrote one *New York Times* reporter, attempting to capture the rather ominous mystique of the place.

Some swore, peering through the black railings to the stone buildings with their arched windows and Corinthian columns, that the whole place was haunted. Stories still were told of the "Bellevue Black Bottle" of the late nineteenth century, containing a mysterious potion supposedly used to winnow out the poorest patients. And of the morgue there where, after a disaster, the bodies literally overflowed. In 1911 the Triangle Shirtwaist Factory building on Washington Square had burned; more than one hundred young seamstresses had died; their blackened bodies had been stacked like cordwood on the piers behind the hospital. Mothers from the Gas House district, the gritty, crime-ridden neighborhood just south of the hospital, used its name to threaten troublesome children; "I'll send ye to Bellevue" was almost as dreaded a warning as "I'll tell the Gerry Society on ye," the nickname of the city's Society for Prevention of Cruelty to Children, hated for its relentless policing tactics.

The hospital's famed psychopathic ward, home to the lunatics, the crazies, the suicidal, and the homicidal, only added to the rumors. Its windows were barred; ivy climbed the stone walls — in the winter, their creepers tangled like old bones. Passersby swore, swore that at night they could hear screams through the glass, see shadows stalking past the windows like unchained beasts.

The current head of that ward, an alienist

named Menas Gregory, had been trying for years to change that haunted reputation. He angrily defended people in his care, many of whom had been brought in against their will when their families had them declared crazy. The lost occupants of his ward needed help, Gregory argued, not mockery, not groundless fear. He worried at how slowly people accepted that, even in his own institution. "There is, at the present time, no place where these patients may receive proper treatment."

Unlike many late-night arrivals to the psychopathic ward, though, Mors seemed happy enough to be there, Gregory told the police. They'd let him bring a pile of books — he was teaching himself better English — and he spent most of his time lying on his cot, reading, muttering over pronunciations. At the end of ten days, Gregory agreed that Mors was "not well mentally." The man was definitely watchful, possibly a little paranoid. He seemed usually controlled, quiet, and polite. Mors was cold, calculating, and somehow just off, slightly inhuman in his reactions. But the alienist saw no evidence that their self-confessed murderer was delusional; it was extremely unlikely that he'd invented the killings; and he wouldn't call him a homicidal lunatic.

Did that make him capable of planning multiple killings? The Bellevue experts could offer a definitive yes. Did that give the district attorney the proof he wanted? A definitive no.

Yes, no, maybe, all the answers led them nowhere, nowhere they wanted to be in a criminal investigation involving eight suspicious deaths. The Mors investigators weren't the only ones stumbling their way through poison murders, but it wasn't particularly comforting to realize that. If anything, a newly published survey only made their situation seem worse.

That same January the city government had released a report declaring that thanks to ill-informed, corrupt, and occasionally drunken coroners, murderers in New York were escaping justice in record numbers. Infanticide, for instance, was almost never punished. And "skillful poisoning can be carried on almost with impunity."

The report was conducted by the city's commissioner of accounts, a reform-minded zealot named Leonard Wallstein. The commissioner had spent a full year studying the long-established political coroner system and concluded that it was a joke, a travesty, a disgrace, a public scandal, and a sheer waste of taxpayers' money. That was only the beginning of his list of epithets. He could add specific complaints about the coroner now in office, Patrick Riordan, who had been observed sneaking nips from his hip flask during recent criminal trials. Two Manhattan civic clubs were demanding Riordan's removal from office.

But Wallstein's report, released in January 1915, was less concerned with the bad habits of one city coroner than with the failures of the whole system. The problems originated, he argued, in the fact that the coroner was an elected official. In New York City, political party bosses regularly fixed elections to reward loyal supporters with lucrative positions. The most powerful political machine in the state belonged to the Democratic Party, which kept headquarters in a rather modest three-story brick building named Tammany Hall, situated on East 14th Street. The party bosses had occupied that home for so long — it was built in 1830 — that many New Yorkers referred to the party machine itself as Tammany Hall.

The political masterminds on East 14th Street had not put the clean government crusader Leonard Wallstein into power. Nor had Tammany Hall wanted him there. In a rare act of rebellion, city voters in 1914 had elected a mayor promising government reform. Wallstein's coroner investigation — prompted in part by the actions of Patrick Riordan — fulfilled a promise made by the administration of Mayor John Purroy Mitchel. One of Mitchel's friends had become entangled in a scheme involving kickbacks between an undertaker and the coroner's department.

The coroner system was only one example of the party machine's bad influence, Wallstein said, but a particularly egregious one. Riordan, who held his position solely through Tammany Hall influence, was only the most obvious symptom of the system's ills. The commissioner estimated that the city spent $172,000 annually on "unqualified coroners, their mediocre physicians and their personal clerks, who spend most of their time on private affairs," or on lining their pockets.

In addition to drawing their salaries, coroners worked on commission. They could — and usually did — bill the city for every body they examined; one assistant coroner "investigated" the same drowning victim more than a dozen times, claiming each time that it had bobbed up at a different location on the Hudson River. Coroners had been known to allow families to claim bodies only if they agreed to let a certain funeral home, which paid a kickback, handle the arrangements. Coroners had other sources of income as well. They sold fake death certificates and thereby covered up murders, criminal abortions, and suicides. One of Wallstein's favorite examples involved a man who had been found dead in his bed, with a bullet wound in his mouth and a revolver in his right hand. The gun contained three loaded cartridges and one exploded one. The coroner gave the cause of death as "rupture of thoracic aneurism."

The city required no medical background or training for coroners, even though they were charged with determining cause of death. The list of New York City coroners, from 1898 to 1915, included eight undertakers, seven politicians, six real estate dealers, two saloonkeepers, two plumbers, a lawyer, a printer, an auctioneer, a wood carver, a carpenter, a painter, a butcher, a marble cutter, a milkman, an insurance agent, a labor leader, and a musician. It also included seventeen physicians, but these, Wallstein pointed out, were men like Patrick Riordan, doctors who had lost their practice and turned to a political position. None of them were asked to pass a test in order to hold office, or exhibit any knowledge of the profession.

As a result, Wallstein found, death certificates were filled out with no effort at determining cause. Among the entries were "could be suicide or murder," and "either assault or diabetes." In one instance a coroner had attributed a death to "diabetes, tuberculosis or nervous indigestion." A few death certificates simply read "act of God." This was not, of course, a uniquely New York problem. A survey by the National Research Council concluded that the average coroner anywhere in the United States was an "untrained and unskilled individual, popularly elected to an obscure office for a short term, with a staff of mediocre ability and inadequate equipment." The research council recommended that all coroner systems be abolished: "It is an anachronistic institution which has conclusively demonstrated its incapacity to perform the functions customarily required of it."

In his own jurisdiction, Wallstein asked the health department to analyze eight hundred cases, randomly chosen from piles of coroner reports. The doctors there discovered that almost half the certificates were so random in their conclusions, or so wrong, that "there is a complete lack of evidence to justify the certified cause of death." Some coroners didn't bother to fill out death certificates at all, just signing them and turning them in. Even so, the health department reported it had waited three years for some certificates to be filed.

Not surprisingly, Wallstein discovered that the city's district attorneys often tried to avoid working with coroners, since these "bungling" so-called experts could easily undermine a prosecution. No wonder, he wrote, that poisoners and other criminals had it so easy in the year 1915. One might expect to find poor equipment and poorly educated criminal investigators in a small village, he added, but "New York City is compelled to get along virtually without aid from the science of legal medicine, a situation which exists in no other great city of the world."

In retrospect, the Mors case illustrated his points almost perfectly.

The suspect claimed that he'd been able to kill some of his chosen victims in just a few minutes. But the coroner had informed the prosecutor that that couldn't be true, that it took at least ten minutes for chloroform to kill a person. Based on that information, the prosecutor hesitated to believe the confession.

Yet the scientific journals supported Mors's confession. One study of 52 chloroform deaths, done only a few years earlier, found that four people had died in less than a minute, and 22 of them had died in less than five minutes.

The coroner also assured the prosecutor that there was no way to find chloroform in a corpse, especially after a burial. Based on this information, the district attorney had refused to exhume a single body. Instead, he declared that it was impossible to find even a full quart of chloroform in a dead body, that an autopsy was a waste of time since it would yield no evidence.

Again, the existing science said almost exactly the opposite. "Chloroform not only withstands but also impedes putrefaction," said a leading toxicology book. In animals killed with chloroform, the compound could be detected in their tissues at least four weeks after death; in the brain, where it tended to concentrate, it could be found months after death. Further, the burying of a body tended to prevent the volatile compound from evaporating.

Contrary to the confusion created by the Rice trial, toxicologists were clear that chloroform was definitely an irritant. People who swallowed chloroform — and lived to tell the tale — were shocked by the burn in the mouth. Autopsies showed that chloroform left the mucous membranes of the mouth, stomach, and intestines reddened and inflamed. The poison was caustic enough that the skin lining the throat and pharynx was visibly softened, easily peeling loose at just a light touch of a pathologist's gloved fingers.

And whether chloroform was inhaled or swallowed, it left a betraying signature: it darkened the blood and caused it to gather in the brain, lungs, liver, and kidneys, producing clumps of bulbous, overfull blood vessels. Chloroform victims could be slightly yellow in color, showing signs of jaundice, due to the poison's ability to wreak havoc in the liver. Alcoholics, with their often damaged livers, were among those most quickly killed by chloroform; they had been among the most frequent deaths under surgical anesthesia.

Reasonable tests for chloroform in human tissue existed even at the time of Rice's death and had been even better established by 1915. The following directions were available in the 1890s: a chemist should mince tissue, distill it with steam, then boil the resulting "syrup" with a mix of lye and benzene. If chloroform existed in the hot chemical soup, the liquid turned yellowish-red, fluorescing — according to the textbooks — to a "beautiful" yellowish-green if exposed to ultraviolet light.

Other chemical tests could separate the poison into its basic constituents. A basic chloroform molecule consists of five atoms — one of carbon, one of hydrogen, and three of chlorine — clustered neatly together. If a chemist heated some minced tissue and added a destructive element — say, hydrochloric acid — he could gradually break the poison apart, separating the chlorine from the rest of the solution, a process that would confirm the presence of chloroform.

The Bronx coroner obviously didn't know this science, and if he sought advice from colleagues elsewhere in New York City, they were uninformed as well. But the possibility of chemical detection did actually exist in that frozen February when Frederic Mors walked into a police station to boast of murder. If anyone had bothered to look for it.

The police found these scientific excuses infuriating. They believed that Mors was the murderer he claimed to be.

The sheriff had said so publicly, infuriating the district attorney. In a press conference the prosecutor conceded that it was "probable" that Mors had "hurried the deaths" of eight people, maybe more — the police had discovered that another nine deaths at the home appeared suspicious. But probability wasn't proof, and as they had no eyewitnesses, a suspect with diagnosed paranoid tendencies, and absolutely no evidence of poison in any of the bodies, the prosecutor decided that he could not justify taking the case to court.

The Bronx district attorney stated: "Mors' fellow employees and others have given circumstantial evidence, they have told of deaths under suspicious circumstances, they have even told of smelling the odor of chloroform about Mors' person, but nothing they have said would be accepted by a judge or jury as proof of the fact that a crime had been committed in the manner described by Mors."

The prosecutor's office had released the Odd Fellows home superintendent from custody, citing lack of evidence that he conspired to eliminate residents in his care. But officials couldn't quite bring themselves to let go of Mors. The district attorney made some calls, pulled some strings, and —

ignoring the report from Bellevue that found him less than certifiable — had the suspected killer committed to an asylum, hoping to use the fact that he had been institutionalized as just cause to deport him back to Austria.

Mors was sent to the Hudson River State Hospital for the Insane in Poughkeepsie. He had been there about three months when he learned of the deportation plan. A week before his scheduled removal, in May 1915, Mors walked away from the asylum — simply disappeared on a warm spring day. In response to an angry complaint, the director of the hospital pointed out that the asylum wasn't a home for the criminally insane and that he'd been given no warnings about Mors when he'd admitted him. The staff hadn't considered him dangerous. His behavior had been what it was at Bellevue — polite, quiet, and maybe a little "paranoically inclined," as Gregory had put it. But no one at the asylum had thought that he might be someone to keep locked away.

Mors disappeared so completely that the police suspected that he'd once again changed his name. He'd been born in Austria with the name Milnarik. He'd explained the change carefully in that first confession, as he watched the detectives through the haze of cigarette smoke. He'd picked the new name for its meaning in Latin. It meant Death.

By the time Frederic Mors disappeared with the spring winds, the city and state governments had come to grim agreement. "It is clear," Leonard Wallstein told the New York newspapers, "that the welfare of the city absolutely requires the immediate abolition of the elective coroner's system . . ."

The governor, embarrassed by all the attention being given to corruption in the state's major city, demanded that Riordan step down from office. And the state legislature passed a bill that had been consistently defeated in earlier sessions, establishing a new medical examiner system for New York City. It required that the position be filled by a qualified doctor, one with pathology experience, who would need to pass stringent professional tests to get the job, and who would appoint a well-trained staff, the kind capable of building a case at least against a self-confessed murderer.

The law had one catch, though. The clever politicians of Tammany Hall had built in a three-year delay — the medical examiner system wouldn't become official until January 1918. The authors of the clause expected that by that time, the reformers would be out of office, and the new mayor — well, he would damn well do as he was told.

# TWO:
# WOOD ALCOHOL
# (CH$_3$OH)
## 1918–1919

As he liked to boast — and did, as often as possible — John F. "Red Mike" Hylan was a self-made man.

As a politician, he wangled an amendment to New York's state constitution that created two new judgeships in Brooklyn. Hylan then took one for himself. After all, as he pointed out, he was a fully qualified lawyer. He had worked as a locomotive engineer for the Brooklyn Elevated while studying for his law degree — until he was fired, reportedly for reading textbooks while he drove the train. He did not think affectionately of his old employer. One of his loudly voiced beliefs was that the city needed a public transportation system, free of the greedy railroad bosses. And of course, controlled instead by the party machine.

Tammany Hall considered Hylan a man with potential. People noticed him — big, pink-faced, copper-haired, with a showy mustache and a booming, blustering voice. He was gratifyingly unlike the pedantic reformists running the city, especially the annoyingly preachy Mayor Mitchel. In 1917 the party tapped Hylan to run against Mitchel. The new candidate confidently assured the voters that reformers were intellectual elitists, all talk, no action, filling the city offices with "lazy do-nothings, rolling around in city automobiles with cigars in their mouths and making themselves conspicuous at baseball games when they should be in their offices."

A majority of New York voters agreed. Hylan's election was considered a stunning upset and, by many, a depressing defeat of good government. Even President Woodrow Wilson was startled into impolitic comment, "How is it possible for the greatest city in the world to place such a man in high office?" But Red Mike stepped into the job with triumphant assurance, standing on the white marble steps of City Hall, bareheaded, his hair glowing like a torch in the fall sunlight. "We have had all the reform that we want in this city for some time to come," he announced.

It wasn't just talk. Hylan immediately began restoring the party faithful to office. One of the first was ex-coroner Patrick

Riordan. And while he was mostly successful at restoring the fallen, the mayor would later concede that the Riordan appointment did not go exactly as he had hoped.

The tireless Leonard Wallstein, now representing the newly formed Citizens' Union, promptly threatened legal action. The *New York Times* pointedly recounted Riordan's past in embarrassing detail, including the misconduct hearings where "witness after witness testified that Riordan was incompetent and was repeatedly intoxicated while on duty."

Angry civic groups reminded Hylan — and the public — that Riordan lacked even the most basic qualifications written into the law, which specified "a skilled microscopist and pathologist." Riordan had not even pretended to abide by the new law, which required that he take a civil service examination for the position. Further, three well-trained doctors, all with backgrounds in pathology, *had* applied and passed the examination: Dr. Otto Schultz, a professor of medical jurisprudence at Columbia University; Dr. Douglas Symmers, a professor of pathology at New York University; and Dr. Charles Norris, chief of laboratories at Bellevue and Allied Hospitals.

Hylan had not foreseen such energetic opposition. He'd already ordered new, gold-leaf letters put on the doors of every coroner's office in the five boroughs, each reading "Dr. Patrick J. Riordan, Chief Medical Examiner." The new mayor didn't care for being pushed around by a bunch of outsiders. He decided to show his critics who was boss by punishing the overqualified applicants. The mayor's office announced that by taking the required examination, all three of those applicants had engaged in criminal behavior.

The reasoning went thus: the doctors had been required to perform autopsies as part of the examination. But state law specified that unclaimed bodies were to go to medical schools for teaching purposes. Since the job applicants had prevented that process, the mayor said, he was directing the civil service commission to file felony charges against them. The three doctors might have to do jail time, he warned, which would bar them from holding the city office.

In late January the accused applicants, a trio in dark suits and stony expressions, stood in a city courtroom. There they had an unobstructed view of the Hylan-appointed civil service commission consulting with Patrick Riordan, who could be seen nodding his white head during a whispered discussion. According to published accounts of the meeting, the head of the civil service commission then leaned forward and addressed each physician: "Doctor, you are accused of a felony in that you performed an autopsy illegally and you are asked to show cause why your name should not be stricken from the civil service list. Have you anything to say?" The applicants refused to cooperate. All three replied that they first wanted the charges set out in writing. They had been given no explanation of why they were facing criminal charges for taking a city-required test. The civil service commission's allegation that they were guilty of "infamously disgraceful conduct" did not constitute a legal complaint, according to their attorneys, who stood beside them.

Fine, then. The commission postponed the hearing, announcing that all would return once the formal charges were drafted. But before the hearing could be rescheduled, even before the week was out, Wallstein led a blast of renewed protests that pushed the state government to intervene. Republican Governor Charles S. Whitman, a former Manhattan district attorney, informed Hylan that his actions were in violation of the law, which did indeed require a qualified forensic scientist for the position, and that his tactics were an embarrassment to the state and "an offense against public decency." Whitman informed the mayor that he wanted to see a professional medical examiner in New York City — immediately.

On January 31, 1918, Hylan appointed Bellevue's Charles Norris as the new medical examiner. He had warm feelings, he insisted, for his new agency head. All he had ever wanted was "a high-class man for this post." In reality, the choice of Norris was a small but bitter act of rebellion. Norris had been ranked second in the examination results, behind the professor from Columbia. Hylan couldn't justify dropping to the third choice, but he refused to be pushed all the way. To emphasize that point, he announced that Norris should consider himself on probation for the next three months.

But Norris took a six-month leave from his job in the Bellevue laboratory anyway. He knew he was in.

It would be imprecise to say that Dr. Charles Norris loved the job of chief medical examiner. He lived it and breathed it. He spent his own money on it. He gave it power and prominence and wore himself into exhaustion and illness over it. Under his direction, the New York City medical examiner's office would become a department that set forensic standards for the rest of the country. And Norris himself would become something of a celebrity, described by *Time* magazine as the "famed, sardonic, goat-bearded, public spirited" medical examiner who "battled for pure food laws, fought against quack doctors, Prohibition, unsanitary restaurants, pronounced on many a suicide and murder that perplexed police, made his name and detective work known in medico-legal circles the world over."

The key term in that exuberant, lengthy description, the reason Norris accepted one of the most spectacularly reluctant job offers in the city's history, could be found in those two words "public spirited." Journalists tended to emphasize the public side of Norris's personality — the outsize former-college-football-player build, the buoyant laugh and quick wit, the dramatic face with its intense dark eyes and lowering eyebrows — and gloss over the intense sense of purpose that really defined the man.

Everyone knew that Norris didn't have to work for the money. His father, Joseph Parker Norris, was a descendant of the merchant banker family that had founded Norristown, Pennsylvania; his mother, Frances Stevens Norris, was a daughter of the first president of the Bank of Commerce in New York City. Born on December 4, 1867, in Hoboken, New Jersey, Norris began his schooling at Cutler's Private School, a tony little Manhattan institution founded by the Harvard-educated tutor of Theodore Roosevelt. He then went to Yale University, where he earned a bachelor of philosophy with an emphasis on science; from there he went to Columbia University's College of Physicians and Surgeons, where he received his doctorate in medicine in 1892. He then studied abroad, first at a series of medical schools in Germany, then in Vienna, where he decided to specialize in pathology and bacteriology. He returned to New York in 1896 and took a job as a pathology lecturer at Columbia. In 1904 he left to become director of the main laboratory at Bellevue and Allied Hospitals.

People would forget, as Norris assumed the mantle of public crime fighter, how much he enjoyed basic medical research. While at Columbia and Bellevue, he published paper after paper on infectious disease: "The Bactericidal Action of Lymph Taken from the Thoracic Duct of the Dog," "Spirochetal Infection of White Rats,"

"Influence of Fasting on the Bactericidal Action of the Blood," "Anterior Poliomyelitis," "Detection of Typhoid Carriers," and even "Red Leg in Frogs," an analysis of an extremely nasty bacterial infection that broke blood vessels apart, staining once-green limbs red.

As fascinating as the research could be, it barely tapped Norris's reservoir of energy or his capacity for public service. He'd been brought up in the tradition: his childhood had steeped him in stories of his ancestors' contributions to their country. Eighteenth-century Norris family members fought in the Revolutionary War, even stripped the lead gutters and rain spouts from their Philadelphia home to make bullets for the Continental Army. His banker grandfather, John Austin Stevens, had negotiated the first loan of $100 million to allow the federal government to finance the Civil War.

In an essay on forensic medicine, Norris would muse on the need for doctors and scientists to lend their talents to criminal investigation, even if it meant less lucrative employment: "A much neglected field of medical endeavor is open to those of us who pursue this widely important branch." What would happen if researchers didn't contribute to the field? he asked, and answered:

"Grave injustice to the relatives of the deceased . . . justice [would be] flaunted and innocent people bear the brunt due to a system which fosters ignorance, prejudice and graft."

It helped that Charles Norris, however high-minded he could sound, also possessed a lively sense of the ridiculous. "We call this the Country Club," he would tell visitors gravely, gesturing them into his departmental offices, furnished with items from the motley collection left him by Patrick Riordan.

Norris had saved, with some enjoyment, the old coroner's original inventory, which had listed, in bitterly meticulous detail: three (dented, according to Riordan's notes) brass cuspidors, one curio closet (glass front intact), one safe (large), two telephone booths, four rugs, thirty-one chairs (two broken, one destroyed), eleven rolltop desks (one in bad shape), three wooden file cabinets, two clocks, one fan, one costumer (or coat rack), and four wooden wardrobes (one in several pieces). The rugs (filthy), they'd thrown away. One slightly blood-spattered carpet from a murder investigation was eventually salvaged to cover the floor of the Country Club lounge.

Norris at least had a new home for his department's offices and laboratories: in Bellevue's recently completed pathology building. Standing a stately six stories, solid with granite, dressed up by long arched windows, the building had been designed with the intention of coordinating the city's forensic services. Here the city morgue was located, as well as the laboratories and autopsy rooms used by pathologists to study the dead. There was plenty of room for the medical examiner's offices and, to Norris's delight, some spare space on the third floor for a forensic chemistry laboratory, something which he was determined to establish.

As he wrote to Mayor Hylan, the location benefited them all. Riordan may have handed over all his battered furnishings, but he had left behind not a scrap of laboratory equipment. It made sense that "the place for the laboratory force of the medical examiner's office should be where its seat of greatest activity resided." Further, as Norris reminded the mayor, Bellevue offered the doctors working for him free access to the glassware, instruments, and chemicals of the pathology department.

The resentful mayor had cut the medical examiner's budget by some $65,000 from what he had offered Riordan. Norris responded by constantly needling the mayor for more money — and by paying for needed supplies himself. He'd inherited a comfortable income, and throughout his tenure he used it to make sure his department was adequately equipped. His first purchase, out of personal funds, was laboratory equipment needed to test for bacterial infections.

He'd assembled a capable staff in his Manhattan office, which would handle major lab work for all the boroughs. He kept a couple of physicians on and brought in some new pathologists, notably a fiercely intelligent Harlem doctor named Thomas Gonzales. He worried, though, about the staff he'd inherited in Brooklyn, Queens, and the Bronx. The doctors there seemed lazy to him. Norris warned the mayor that he might have to replace a certain amount of "useless timber." But first he'd see how they responded to new standards. It surprised no one who knew Charles Norris that he had plans, lots of them. He would develop new rules for handling bodies. He would hire someone to run the chemistry lab, clerks to answer the phones, and stenographers to take and type notes on all bodies processed by the laboratory. He would create files on each case and insist that medical examiner employees, when testifying in court, refer to the recorded information rather than "memory," as in the past.

"This work, which I may term 'organization,' " has apparently not been tried before, Norris wrote to Hylan, displaying his contempt for the previous system. The relaxed environment of the old coroner's office, he promised the mayor, was now a thing of the past.

By April, Norris was happily harassing other city departments. He complained to the district attorney's office that his men were kept standing about in the courtroom halls for hours, waiting to be called for testimony. He complained to the police department that the stations weren't stocked with soap and towels for the medical examiners to use before and after handling bodies.

"I wish to call to your attention the delay of the police precincts in their notification of homicides to the office of the Chief Medical Examiner," he wrote to the police commissioner. For example, he'd been notified of a shooting on the Upper West Side some two hours after the police had reached the crime scene. It was the second time this had happened since Norris had taken office. In this case no real harm had been done, but "in many cases, I can conceive very well that non-attendance on the part of the Chief Medical Examiner or his assistants might be detrimental to the criminal investigation of a case." He asked that desk lieutenants in police precincts be instructed to automatically call his office whenever a homicide or suspicious death occurred.

He wrote to the Bronx district attorney, reporting that certain police officers seemed to be taking bribes to conceal murders. In one case, they'd asked him to declare a suicide; when he'd refused, they'd tried to get an independent doctor to issue the death certificate. "It is entirely out of the question, in my opinion, to even consider the possibility of a suicide on account of the number and situation of the bullet wounds. There were four bullet wounds sprayed across the corpse." How, Norris asked, could the man have accomplished shooting himself in the heart, the shoulder, the leg, and the arm? That might have been the old way of issuing death certificates, but those times were over, and he wanted everyone to know it.

He wrote to hospitals asking them to be quicker in getting bodies to the morgue for examination — one woman's body arrived eight hours after she died. Norris called that completely unacceptable. He insisted that hospitals fill out forms issued by his office for every suspicious death, every detail according to his careful direction. "Your peremptory order," began one response from a ruffled hospital director.

He was even tougher, though, on assistant medical examiners who failed to follow his instructions. He wanted key organs removed at autopsy for chemical analysis — the stomach, for instance, in a suspected poison case — had to be put in a sterile glass jar, labeled, dated, and placed in a sanitary fiber bag. All such evidence would go directly to the chemistry laboratory at Bellevue's pathology building.

Norris wrote to the Brooklyn office demanding meticulous and thorough work in every detail. An assistant medical examiner there had declared a man dead of kidney damage due to use of a salve containing mercury. He'd done so based on a discussion with the man's doctors, but without removing the kidneys for analysis or gathering any other evidence. "Did you make any efforts to procure the salve in order to determine that there *was* mercury?" Norris wrote angrily. When the doctor in question didn't improve fast enough to suit him, Norris fired him.

He chastised personnel in the Bronx office with equal vigor. Norris was particularly exasperated by a report that loosely blamed a man's death on wood alcohol. The document stated that the victim had been drinking heavily in the hours before his collapse. He'd also been stricken with sudden blindness (a classic symptom of wood alcohol poisoning) several hours before lapsing into a coma. The death certificate listed wood alcohol poisoning as a "more than probable" cause.

But "more than probable" was hardly a professional opinion, Norris said. The doctors should have removed liver and brain and preserved them for testing so that the diagnosis could be confirmed. Other evidence — such as the bottle containing the allegedly poisonous whiskey — should have been also saved and analyzed. Witnesses should have been questioned and statements taken down. Without such work, he emphasized, the district attorney had no way to prosecute vendors of liquors containing wood alcohol.

And that mattered, because getting it right had to be the everyday standard of the medical examiner's office. It also mattered because Norris had a worrying idea based on rising numbers of wood alcohol deaths.

He thought the city was looking at the start of a serious health problem. The latest research findings of his newly hired forensic chemist, Alexander Gettler, reinforced his concern. Gettler, a cigar-smoking gambling enthusiast from Brooklyn, possessed none of Norris's aristocratic background but shared his perfectionistic ideals, and, in the case of wood alcohol, his sense of alarm.

Born in 1883, the son of a Hungarian immigrant who had left the country for better opportunities, Gettler learned early to love the magic of chemistry. By the time he graduated from high school, he was hooked by the puzzle of fitting one molecule to another, by the kaleidoscope of colors that glowed in a test tube. His family had no money to send him to college, so he paid for it himself. While working as a ticket agent on the 39th Street Brooklyn-to-Battery ferry, he earned a science degree from the College of the City of New York. To earn his master's at Columbia University, he arranged to work the midnight-to-eight ferry shift. That way he could do homework during the ferry's quiet night hours and attend classes during the day.

Awarded his master's in 1910, Gettler took a job as a chemistry instructor at Bellevue Medical School, then went to work on his doctorate. Two years later Gettler received his Ph.D. from Columbia and was promoted to assistant professor in the medical school. He married a young schoolteacher, Alice Gorman, despite the loud opposition of her Irish Catholic family. Gettler, the Jewish immigrant, simply charmed away their objections, agreeing to move in with his in-laws, taking the top floor of their Brooklyn home. He even attended Sunday services with his wife. "He refused to do confession though," his daughter-in-law would recall years later.

Gettler was not an imposing figure in the style of Charles Norris. A slight man, he had a thin, intense face, serious dark eyes, and carefully smooth dark hair. He was shy with strangers, indifferent to politics, and impatient with the constant journalistic interest in his work. With nosy reporters, he usually retreated behind an annoyingly pedantic facade: "A personality as colorless as the sodium chloride [table salt, NaCl] that he works with," wrote one frustrated reporter, after a series of dust-dry responses to questions.

That image made people who knew Gettler laugh. He liked viciously competitive bowling, the nosebleed seats at baseball games, and any and all horse races, as long as he could place a bet. He called his bookie from his office every week. He talked Alice into vacationing at the Saratoga racetrack. He never could resist a good card game, playing weekly with fellow gamblers from the office. His wife joked that the real reason he had moved into her family's house was so that she'd have company when he was out with the boys.

Gettler brought that competitive streak directly into the laboratory. He hated to give up on a chemical analysis, and he positively hated the idea that some poisoner off the street could outwit him. He was such a good chemist that Bellevue had refused to turn him loose from its pathology work. Further, he genuinely enjoyed the teaching work he was doing for NYU. So if Norris wanted Gettler to work for him — and he definitely did — he had to settle for a joint appointment.

It would be a challenge, Norris warned his new hire. No other city in the United States had a dedicated toxicology laboratory. Gettler would have to design the lab from scratch and invent a methodology for the New York office. There were no training programs in forensic toxicology; there were astonishingly few books on the subject, most of them based on European research.

In the days of coroners like Patrick Riordan, high-profile poisoning cases in New York had been sent to chemistry professors at the city's well-respected universities. And they had often done good work. But as Gettler noted, those chemists "had but little experience in toxicological analyses of human organs" and little time to spend on the work itself, usually squeezing it in around other demands. In one case, a professor had taken twenty months to analyze some organs (during which time he had taken a three-month vacation to Europe).

In other words, the job — uncharted and overwhelming — was perfect for Gettler, a man who liked to cram as much work as possible into his hours, loved to juggle multiple challenges, and believed passionately in the power of chemistry. He took a straightforward approach. If a test didn't exist, he would invent it. If research methods didn't exist, he would develop them himself. If a new poison or drug came on the market, he went off to a butcher shop, just around the corner from his Brooklyn home, and bought three pounds of liver. He would arrive at Bellevue carrying his twine-wrapped and bloodstained parcel under his arm. In his laboratory, he would slice the liver into neat segments, inject each with a different drug, and grind up the organ pieces. He would then experiment with different ways of extracting the injected chemicals from the tissue, looking for ways to detect ever smaller and smaller amounts of each poison.

It was a rough beginning, a bloody one, and a messy one, but he had to start somewhere.

Gettler used his liver test mostly on newly invented poisons, the ones that he anticipated could someday be a problem. For the familiar, everyday toxins, he could often obtain a body for study instead. In the case of wood alcohol, for example, Gettler could now, unfortunately, count on a steady supply of cadavers from the morgue.

Wood alcohol — technically known as methyl alcohol, but also as wood spirit, hydroxymethane, carbinol, colonial spirit, Columbian spirit, and, some years later, methanol — was in itself nothing new. The ancient Egyptians had used it in their embalming processes. For centuries it had been the essential ingredient in homemade whiskey. Its chemical formula had been identified in 1661 by a chemist who called it "spirit of box" because he'd made it by distilling boxwood. The term *methyl* was derived from the Greek *methy* (meaning wine) and *hyle* (meaning wood, or, more precisely, patch of trees).

The chemical structure of wood alcohol is simple: three hydrogen atoms bonded to a single carbon atom (in a cluster known as a methyl group), with one oxygen atom and another hydrogen atom tagging along. It is also simple to make, as industrialists and moonshiners had realized, requiring little more than wood and heat. The process was called destructive distillation. Slabs and slices of wood went into a closed container and were heated to at least 122 degrees Fahrenheit (50 degrees centigrade). As the wood cooked into charcoal, its natural liquids vaporized. That vapor could be cooled, condensed, and distilled into a rather murky soup containing methyl alcohol, acetone, and acetic acid. A second distilling would separate out the pure methyl alcohol, a liquid as clear as glass and as odorless as ice, from the other ingredients.

By the end of the nineteenth century, manufacturing plants called wood factories were clustered along the East Coast, more than forty in Pennsylvania alone. The factories burned thousands of trees a year, mostly birch, beech, maple, oak, elm, and alder, to fill a near-endless appetite for charcoal and wood by-products. Methyl alcohol could be used as a solvent, to make varnish, as an ingredient in dyes, and as a fuel. Some countries, such as England and Germany, prohibited its use in domestic products, considering it too risky. But the United States allowed it into a host of household materials, including essence of peppermint, lemon extract, cologne, after-shaves such as citrus-scented Florida water or bay rum, and liniments such as witch hazel.

It was also used to "denature" grain alcohol, which essentially meant changing drinkable spirits into a lethal industrial product. Methyl alcohol was so poisonous — an estimated two tablespoons could kill a child — that one needed only a little to turn drinking alcohol into a toxic substance. The resulting "industrial" alcohol was exempt from government liquor taxes but was also required by law to be labeled as a poison.

Long before Gettler arrived as city toxicologist, wood alcohol had achieved a sinister reputation. It was mountain alcohol, cheap street alcohol, and everyone knew that it could, and did, kill its share of unlucky drinkers. But at this particular moment Gettler suspected — no, he was positive — that the reputation of wood alcohol was destined to get worse.

"The prohibition by our government of the manufacture of distilled liquors will unquestionably lead to much 'moonshining,' adulteration and dilution of liquors offered to the public," he predicted in a 1918 article in the *Journal of the American Medical Association*.

Prohibition hovered just a legislative breath away when Gettler made his report. The Eighteenth Amendment to the U.S. Constitution, which would prohibit the manufacture, sale, transportation, import, and export of "intoxicating liquors," had passed both houses of Congress in December 1917. A full thirty-six states were needed to ratify the amendment to make it law. Within a year fifteen states approved the measure, and the Ohio-based Anti-Saloon League and the Women's Christian Temperance Union were demanding that the rest of the country fall into line.

The Anti-Saloon League, the most powerful of those lobbying groups, had sent its best political organizer to New York City, which it liked to call "the liquor center of

America." The league routinely cited federal records showing that in one week city residents consumed some 75,000 quarts of gin, 76,000 quarts of brandy, 500 quarts of absinthe, and more than 500,000 quarts of beer, wine, and miscellaneous spirits. That unrestricted guzzling of alcohol was about to stop, organizer William Anderson promised. "I'm willing to work night and day," he said. "We won't admit defeat."

With such promises — or threats — occurring daily, Gettler suspected that the city's equally dedicated drinkers were already bracing against the disappearance of legal alcohol. They were building secret stills and stockpiling supplies. "That such is the case even at this early period is quite evident from the recent poisoning in this city of over thirty persons, six of whom died," he wrote. The whiskey that killed them contained "a considerable amount of wood alcohol."

Wood alcohol came wonderfully cheap — a few cents a glass. It could be distilled out of discarded wood chips, sawdust, lumber scrap, bits and pieces of dead plants — and it tasted just fine going down. "The refined wood alcohol tastes like ethyl [grain] alcohol and, moreover is considerably cheaper," Gettler wrote, "hence the adulterator buys the latter, ignorant that severe poisoning, blindness and often death lurk within it."

Why is one alcohol so poisonous when another — spirits made from grain — is so much safer? It has to do with the way wood alcohol's chemistry interacts with human metabolic processes. As the body's enzymes break apart the carbon, hydrogen, and oxygen that form the alcohol, those atoms form new and more dangerous breakdown products. The deadly chemical detritus consists mostly of formaldehyde and formic acid. Methyl alcohol is toxic in its own right, as Gettler noted, but formic acid is at least six times more deadly. Further, methyl alcohol metabolizes comparatively slowly, lingering in the body. The conversion to the "more dangerous poisons" can take up to five days, meaning that the wood alcohol drinker can stew in an increasingly lethal cocktail for the better part of a week.

Gettler wanted doctors to be aware of, and to watch for, the pattern of a wood alcohol death: a sudden sense of weakness, severe abdominal pain and vomiting, blindness, a slip into unconsciousness, heart failure. He wanted them to brace for the onset of Prohibition, which ensured new and more dangerous alcohol issues. Both he and Norris anticipated a dramatic rise in wood alcohol deaths.

Neither man was persuaded by the ideals that supporters of the new amendment expressed. Neither believed that the prohibition of legal alcohol was likely to create a society that suddenly rejected the pleasures of beer, wine, and cocktails. Rather, "we feel it timely to warn physicians, coroners and health officers in order that they may be on their guard" and anticipate an epidemic of wood alcohol poisoning.

Gettler's message to doctors was simple: *This is poison. Warn everyone. Do it now.*

Poison was already in the air that spring of 1918, both figuratively and literally. It tracked through the newspaper headlines in a litany of horror stories–dying children, blinded villagers, dead and disfigured soldiers.

The United States had declared war on Germany in April 1917, joining the Great War. The first American soldiers arrived in France that June; a month later Germany launched the war's most spectacular poison gas attack, bombarding the battlefield at Ypres with bright yellow shells loaded with mustard gas. In November the British captured a stockpile of enemy mustard gas shells (Germany produced more than ten thousand tons of the gas during the war) and returned the attack, bombarding the Kaiser's troops with their own poison bombs.

Mustard gas derives from a thick, oily liquid that takes its color from the sulfur it contains. Mixed with an explosive variety of other chemicals, the liquid — called sulfur mustard — fragments into a brownish-yellow aerosol mist. The "mustard" itself is the point, though; the concentrated sulfur it contains mixes with other ingredients to become a ferocious form of sulfuric acid. Known technically as a vesicant, or blistering agent, it burns on contact, through uniforms, through leather, and through skin, raising a thick layer of oozing yellow blisters, searing the eyes into crusted blindness. If inhaled, mustard gas plasters bloody blisters across the lining of the lungs, making breathing a rasping, painful misery. German military strategists considered it a disabling agent rather than a killer. It was rarely instantly lethal (although scientists would later find it to be a potent carcinogen) but always excruciatingly painful.

Medical personnel, as well as soldiers in their letters home, described the effects of poison gases. "I wish people who talk about going on with this war whatever the cost could see the soldiers suffering from mustard gas poisoning," wrote one nurse, who told of teenage boys strapped down to their beds, fighting for breath, their voices burned away to a hoarse whisper, praying to die.

Although traditional weapons killed far more people in the Great War, poison gas gave a new nightmare edge to the fighting. "The chemists' war," some people nicknamed it, as Germany experimented with other gases, releasing lethal greenish clouds of chlorine; the French introduced phosgene, which combined chlorine and carbon monoxide; and the Americans developed Lewisite — an ugly combination of chlorine and arsenic.

By the summer of 1918 the United States was also manufacturing mustard gas — "the deadliest instrument of warfare yet devised," the New York newspapers called it. The chief army chemist explained that it was the most useful of the gases, because unlike phosgene it didn't break down in sunlight, and unlike Lewisite it was stable when wet. The Germans, it turned out, had first considered cyanide gas, but they'd decided it dispersed too easily in air. That disintegration made its effects mild compared to those of the heavier, oily droplets of mustard gas, which settled in a poisonous blanket over the trenches where soldiers had sought protection.

The United States had hesitated at first to use mustard gas, the military said, because it seemed somehow more akin to torture than other weapons. It might seem peculiar to say that, when men and boys were so routinely blown to bits on the battlefield. But poison seemed a different kind of evil, insidious and cowardly, without the redeeming heroics of combat.

On the home front, New York City — like much of the world in those days — was suffering from another murderous by-product of the war. It could be seen in the new look of the streets, patterned by a blizzard of white masks. Letter carriers, transit workers, train passengers, office and factory workers were wearing, even required to wear, protective masks, not against gas but against the so-called Spanish flu, which seemed to be blowing in from the battlefields.

Influenza was always feared, but this infection spread like a black plague, unreasonably fast, impossibly deadly. The first diagnosed cases in New York, according to the city's public health commissioner, were three sailors from the merchant marine, on leave in Manhattan in mid-September. By

November 1918 the Public Health Service had tallied more than twenty thousand deaths in New York City alone.

The city imposed one rule after another attempting to prevent the infection's spread. Travelers at the railroad stations who appeared ill were stopped on the platform and examined: if they had any flu symptoms, they were banned from public transit. Businesses and factories were ordered on a schedule of staggered opening and closing hours to thin the rush hour crowds. Schools remained open, but children arrived wearing cheesecloth masks and garlic tied around their necks, which their mothers hoped would fend off infection. People were encouraged to avoid large gatherings in theaters, saloons, and dance halls. Theaters were required to open all windows; if police found them shut, the businesses would be closed. Ministers voluntarily suspended church services. The state's Department of Health Services made "unguarded" coughing and sneezing a misdemeanor offense, subject to police detainment.

Yet the influenza continued to spread. Private hospitals, with every bed full, turned people away daily. Public hospitals, like Bellevue, lacked that option, but so many doctors and nurses fell ill that the trustees

debated closing the hospital. Rooms overflowed; cots were crammed into the halls;
when the hospital ran out of rooms, staffers
took doors off their hinges and used them
for dividers. In the pediatric ward, children
were crammed three to a bed. Deaths averaged ten a day at Bellevue; some days they
totaled more than fifty. "It got to the place
where I would only see patients twice," one
intern recalled. "Once when they came in
— and again when I signed the death certificate."

Norris's staff was doing little but processing influenza cases, desperately trying to
record influenza deaths, keep correct numbers, save blood samples, and note deaths
due to other causes. As Norris wrote to the
mayor, the hospital's regular staff was so
busy trying to save a few of the sick that
"they were unable to furnish death certificates to the unfortunate relatives or friends."
Everyone, from physicians to chemists, was
pressed into the hated job of churning out
the certificates. At the same time Norris was
trying to protect his beleaguered staff from
being sent to war. The Selective Service had
gone into effect in mid-September. The war
department had set draft age at 18 to 45,
which meant that eight of Norris's eleven
doctors were eligible.

"Should any of our men be drawn away in the draft, it will be next to impossible to obtain physicians of training in pathology and pathological work in general who could take their place and we cannot get along with a smaller number of physicians," Norris wrote urgently to the army, pointing out that the previous year, his office had handled more than twelve thousand cases, and that had been before the epidemic. "We cannot do the important work which the office must perform" with fewer men.

In particular, Norris wanted to keep his thirty-four-year-old toxicologist from being called up. He wrote another letter, pleasant in tone, edged with an underlying threat. Gettler had done several examinations of "poisons and drugs removed from the clothes of soldiers" in the past year. In fact, the toxicologist "comes in touch with the soldiers and sailors who die within city limits and there have been a considerable number of cases which we have had to handle delicately, and I'm happy to say that were are on the most friendly working basis with the various services of the government."

Norris hoped to keep it that way; no one would enjoy publicizing reports concerning drunken soldiers (such as the one who had recently fallen off a subway platform just as the train arrived) or the several sailors poisoned by wood alcohol. His files contained records of both. The letter turned out to be very convincing or, some might say, an effective kind of blackmail. Either description worked — Norris didn't care. The point was that he got to keep his very necessary chemist, doing his very necessary job.

In Gettler's laboratory, the wooden floorboards were already discolored by chemical drips and sizzles. The white plaster walls were smudged gray by smoke and fumes, and the stone counters were crowded with glass bottles and flasks and dishes of discolored liver samples.

In this room, where the background music was the sizzle of gas burners, the snakelike hiss of distillation, and the bubbling of flasks over flames, poison defined the world outside. To others, the warm glow of a gas-lit window might signify a family evening at home. But here chemists tested blood and tissue for the carbon monoxide that fed those lamps. They worried about the strychnine used in medicinal tonics, the cyanide used in photographic processing, and the arsenic packed into rat baits. As they all knew, here in the third-floor laboratory, the most ordinary of household supplies could be used to kill; in the first month of 1919, Gettler had determined that a thirteen-year-old girl had poisoned a baby simply by using Lysol to clean its bottle.

So it was that as Prohibition moved toward reality — Wyoming had become the thirty-sixth state to ratify the amendment on January 16, 1919 — Gettler and his small staff returned to the idea that wood alcohol was about to increase in popularity. The Eighteenth Amendment, now that it had attained full ratification, was scheduled to go into effect in 1920. Already, though, the medical examiner's office was charting a rise in alcohol poisoning, as New Yorkers hurried to find alternative supplies.

By the late fall of 1919 more than sixty people in the city had died from drinking wood alcohol and another hundred had been blinded. The same pattern played out across the country: 70 wood alcohol deaths in the Connecticut Valley, 9 in Chicago, 15 in Cleveland, and 3 in Memphis; 12 cases of blindness in Denver; and so on. But the official reports underestimated the totals, Norris warned. Many doctors still didn't know how to detect a wood alcohol death — the chemical procedures were still incomplete.

His department hoped to change that.

"During the years 1918 and 1919, I have had occasion to examine over 700 human organs for alcohol," Gettler wrote, in a paper explaining detection of wood alcohol in human tissue. In preparation for the expected deluge of poisoning cases, Gettler — already showing his perfectionist nature — had evaluated fifty-eight different methods for identifying wood alcohol, both in tissue and in the so-called whiskey itself.

He compared the tests' effectiveness on "eight typical good grain whiskies," then on alcoholic cider and five confiscated samples of wood alcohol. He tested them on another five cocktails made by mixing wood alcohol with water: each time he increased the amount of water, diluting the alcohol and making it more difficult to detect.

He then evaluated methods of detecting wood alcohol in human organs. His favorite method involved grinding up a chunk of tissue — 500 grams, about the size and weight of a roll of nickels — and putting the pinkish ooze into a flask with a drop of mineral oil (to prevent frothing). He then steamed his ooze by putting the flask in a boiling water bath, which turned it into a dark sludge. He mixed the sludge with acid and allowed it to cool. If he then stirred an unstable, reactive oxygen compound into the sludge — say, a fizzy salt like potassium dichromate — and reheated the flask, the ever-active oxygen triggered a further breakdown of the alcohol inside. Formaldehyde would come bubbling out. Most alcohols produced only a trace of formaldehyde, but wood alcohol released an overpowering amount — stinging, poisonous, and unmistakable.

Testing a bottle of spirits involved a similarly elaborate process of distillation and oxidation. But Gettler recognized that for inspectors in the field, who needed to do a quick test in a saloon, lugging around a distillation apparatus was awkward, not to say impossible. The on-the-road alternative was to heat a copper coil to red hot and plunge the glowing metal into the alcohol. The heated metal would cause wood alcohol to interact with oxygen in the air — a different kind of oxidation — and release a nose-stinging whiff of formaldehyde.

An inspector had to be willing to risk numbing his sense of smell to conduct the portable test, and the copper wire results were reliable only if the bottle contained a high percentage of wood alcohol, a good 40 proof (i.e., 20 percent) or more. If the wood alcohol was dilute, perhaps used just to spice up other ingredients, "it is extremely difficult, even impossible, for many people to detect the presence of methyl [wood] alcohol," Gettler wrote. "I have tried this experiment on many individuals, using the same liquor, and found that some said methyl alcohol was present, others believed it to be absent, and still others were undecided."

Gettler wasn't fazed by that challenge. When had the detection of poison ever been easy?

The bloody, poisonous, horrible war was finally over — an armistice was signed in 1918, and the official treaty of surrender was concluded at Versailles in 1919. Parades, celebrations, and parties reigned in New York as the troops came spilling off ships.

But Mayor Hylan was not in a celebratory mood. He wrote to Norris and other department heads that diligent city employees should not become overly festive: "My attention has been called to the fact that when transports with returning troops are passing up the river, great quantities of torn papers are thrown . . . City employees should be sufficiently well informed to know that such acts are in violation of the ordinances, and cause additional work and expense to the City, not only in the cleaning up of this illegal litter, but in the waste of paper. Will you kindly issue instructions forbidding this practice?"

And by the way, department heads should stop asking for money to improve their departments. Norris, he'd found, was a particular pest. As Hylan informed his medical examiner, "It is impossible for an official to do any constructive work if he is to be constantly annoyed in this manner."

Norris ignored his complaints. In December, Hylan wrote again to Norris, begging him to stop lobbying for a larger staff. If Norris would give up "playing politics, that is endeavoring to fill positions," the medical examiner would find that he had extra time to work on improving his department from within. But the mayor acknowledged in the same letter that he'd been telling Norris this for two years; he had no real expectation of his advice being taken.

Norris, naturally, continued to demand that larger staff. Meanwhile he and Gettler decided to launch a campaign alerting residents of "the liquor capitol of the country" to the dangers of wood alcohol. "We have found what apparently is an increased number of cases of methyl alcohol, as shown by chemical examination of the viscera," Norris wrote to the health department. "This would indicate that the alcohol sold all over the city contains methyl alcohol in dangerous amounts."

In December there had been forty-two wood alcohol deaths in Manhattan and another nine in the surrounding boroughs; more than a hundred new cases of alcohol-related blindness had also been reported. The National Committee for the Prevention of Blindness, which kept its headquarters on Manhattan's Upper West Side, pointed out that this pattern was repeating across the country. Nearly a thousand people nationwide had recently lost their eyesight due to wood alcohol poisoning. Doctors attributed the blindness to the destructive effect of formic acid on the optic nerves.

As the month wound down, as the official Prohibition date got closer, Norris, Gettler, the city health commissioner, the head of the New York Academy of Medicine, and the Committee for Blindness Prevention held a press conference urging the city to prevent the sale and distribution of wood alcohol and all other forms of methyl alcohol. "One teaspoon of wood alcohol is enough to cause blindness," Norris warned. And drinking a tumbler of the stuff could kill a man within a few hours.

Gettler, Norris, and their comrades unanimously predicted that Prohibition, rather than making alcohol disappear, would instead create "numerous harmful substitutes for whiskey." They made the prediction in December 1919, too early to say whether they would be proved right or whether they were just expressing the dark perspective that came from too many hours of working in Bellevue's pathology building.

# THREE:
# CYANIDES (HCN, KCN, NaCN)

### 1920–1922

Cocktail parties sparkled defiantly through the last chime of the day, to the dreaded first minute of January 20, 1920. With morning would come the official start of Prohibition, so the revelers danced through the night in black-draped rooms featuring open coffins to collect empty bottles. In Times Square, crowds gathered to mourn the stroke of midnight. The dancers and the mourners were shiny in party clothes, somber in mock funeral wear, dressed up with black top hats and smoke-fine veils, just as drunk as they could be. Some stayed into the morning, crowding along Broadway with their whiskey-fed protests. Others slipped away to continue the festivities in private.

It was easy enough to keep the party going. As soon as legal drinking ended, purveyors of illicit alcohol came helpfully forward. As Gettler had predicted, they offered some devastatingly lethal brews. That January poison alcohol deaths rippled across the country: eight in New York City, four dead in a single day in Hartford, two in Toledo, seven in Washington, D.C. Soon the police discovered that murderers had learned to take advantage. In a typical case, barely a month after Prohibition, two men were found dead in Newark, several hours after buying liquor at a Bowery joint. They were thought to be alcohol deaths until a standard chemical analysis of the bodies found they were loaded with potassium cyanide. The killer, whoever he was, was long gone.

Within a year, the once openly rowdy saloons had given way to secretive speakeasies and to bootleggers who would sneak gin to one's door at a delivery rate of two dollars a bottle. "The speakeasies are a remarkable feature of the new American life," wrote one fascinated British visitor.

Every time you go for a drink there is adventure. I suppose it adds to one's pleasure to change into a pirate or a dark character entering a smuggler's cave. You go to locked and chained doors. Eyes are considering you through peepholes in the wooden walls . . . You sign your name in a book and receive a mysterious-looking card with only a number on it. And you are admitted to a back-parlour bar with a long row of loquacious drinkers. There may be a red signal light which can be operated from the door in case of a revenue officer or police demanding entrance.

When the light flashed over the front door, the patrons fled out the back.

By summer's end, a bare half-year into the new amendment, New York officials were already worrying about enforcement. In August a Brooklyn magistrate presided over the trial of a burglar who had broken into a supposedly closed saloon and spent a night guzzling its gin supplies. The judge vented his frustration: "Prohibition is a joke. It has deprived the poor workingman of his beer and it has flooded the country with rat poison." Police department chemists, analyzing the so-called gin in the Brooklyn bar and around the city, reported that much of it was industrial alcohol, redistilled to try to remove the wood alcohol content. The redistilling was not notably successful. The poisonous alcohol remained, and there was more: the chemists had detected traces of kerosene and mercury and disinfectants, including Lysol and carbolic acid, in the beverages. "Drinkers are taking long chances on their health," warned the police commissioner, "if not their lives."

But for the new speakeasy devotees, the risk was part of the fun. Sometimes it was all the fun. It was amusing and exotic, as the British writer noted, to spend time in the dim light and hot jazz of some hidden corner, to experiment with the strange liquids that appeared at the table. Another groggy patron wrote, about a night of clubbing: the bartender "brought me some Benedictine and the bottle was right. But the liqueur was curious — transparent at the top of the glass, yellowish in the middle and brown at the base . . . Oh, what dreams seemed to result from drinking it . . . That is the bane of speakeasy life. You ring up your friend the next morning to find out whether he is still alive."

At the underground clubs, inventive bartenders enjoyed new respect for disguising the taste of the day's alcohol. They created a new generation of cocktails heavy on fruit juices and liqueurs to mix with the bathtub gin, bright and spicy additions to cover the raw sting of the spirits. There was the Bennett Cocktail (gin, lime juice, bitters), the Bee's Knees (gin, honey, lemon juice), the Gin Fizz (gin, lemon juice, sugar, seltzer water), and the Southside (lemon juice, sugar syrup, mint leaves, gin, seltzer water).

At least, those were the kind of drinks served at the city's classier joints — say Jack and Charlie's 21, on 52nd Street. Or Belle Guinan's El Fay Club on West 45th, where the hostess gleamed like a candelabrum and the house band played "The Prisoner's Song" when dry agents were spotted in the crowd. Down in the Bowery, as the police could tell you, the drink of choice was a cloudy cocktail called Smoke, made by mixing water and fuel alcohol. Smoke joints were tucked into the back of paint stores, drugstores, and markets, among the dry goods and the stacked cans. The drink was blessedly cheap — fifteen cents a glass — and just about pure methyl alcohol.

In a bad season, Smoke deaths in the Bowery averaged one a day. Government agents trying to hunt down suppliers of the poor man's cocktail swore that it was served right from cans stenciled with the word POISON — and that people didn't care. They just gambled that it wouldn't kill them and drank it anyway.

As demands for chemical analysis intensified, Norris was infuriated that the Hylan administration remained so stingy regarding his department. The mayor restricted funds every year, as if still holding on to his initial grudge.

In 1922, as Norris noted in yet another letter to the mayor, he had only forty-one employees in his office (compared to sixty-two under Riordan). Annual pay for the doctors working under him averaged less than $4,000 a year. Chemists didn't even get that — by pestering the mayor constantly, he'd finally managed to get Gettler's salary above $3,000 annually.

His own yearly salary was only $6,000; as Norris pointed out, none of the staff got the kind of incomes enjoyed under the old coroner system. But he was angrier still about the lack of basic support for the department as a whole. All new equipment purchased in 1921 had been paid for by Norris himself or by his staff: every test tube, every scalpel, a new scale to weigh tissue samples, a small brass microscope to study tissue damage. All of it. Gettler was dipping into his less-than-generous salary to buy extra chemical supplies and the weekly allotment of raw liver for his experiments.

The medical examiner's office could not possibly do its best work, Norris said, when the city officials failed to recognize the "well known fact that guilt or innocence may rest entirely on the chemical and biological analyses" of evidence at a crime scene. And if anyone doubted that premise, it was about to be painfully proven in a beautiful little hotel in Brooklyn.

The Hotel Margaret glittered like an enormous holiday ornament on the northeastern corner of Orange Street, in Brooklyn's upscale Columbia Heights neighborhood. Built in 1889, according to the colorful plans of local architect Frank Freeman, the hotel was a twelve-story fantasy of limestone, brick, and terra-cotta, with copper balconies and arched rectangular windows that rose to an ornate peaked roof.

In the 1920s, the hotel offered both overnight accommodations — at a pricey twenty dollars a night — and residential apartments. The latter were so popular that the owners had built an annex to house the long-term residents, crafted in the same tones of copper, red, and gold, offering the same delivery of meals by white-coated waiters, the same copper-grilled elevators manned by uniformed porters, and the same nearly invisible maid service. The elegant Hotel Margaret blended seamlessly into the elegant mansions of the Heights.

At least until the day a retired carpet dealer and his wife were found dead on the bathroom floor of their annex apartment.

"Aged Couple Slain Strangely" read the *New York Times* headline on April 27, 1922, reflecting the bafflement of the police investigators. They'd found seventy-five-year-old Fremont M. Jackson and his sixty-year-old wife, Annie, crumpled on the black and white tile of their bathroom. Both were dressed in street clothes. She lay close to the sink, and he just inside the door.

The Jacksons had died badly. Their teeth were clenched, and their lips were stained with a dried bloody froth. Their faces were oddly bluish, and their skin was patterned over with livid red spots. The physician assigned to the case suspected a double suicide, perhaps by swallowing a quick-acting poison.

But investigators found not a trace of poison in the Jacksons' rooms — no container, vial, or bottle — and no mysterious remnants in the bottom of a drinking glass. And the family members described the couple as happy and healthy, insisting that suicide was out of the question. The Jacksons had barely been married a year. After

101

spending years alone, they had both been enjoying the companionship of a second marriage. Annie Jackson's son sent a telegram from his Massachusetts home, proposing that his mother had died of food poisoning and that the shock of finding her body must have killed her husband.

On Norris's order, one of the assistant medical examiners in the Brooklyn office did an autopsy. It hinted at cyanide, which was known to cause a kind of chemical suffocation and would explain the blue look of oxygen deprivation. But cyanide from where? It killed quickly, too quickly for them to have imbibed it elsewhere and then strolled back home. Police searched the apartment again, once more failing to find a trace of the poison.

"Mr. and Mrs. Jackson met their deaths by poisoning, but whether the drug was self-administered or sent to them is impossible just now to determine," the medical examiner's office announced. "The poison might have been administered in food or drink." The doctor conducting the autopsy had removed both stomachs, placed them in specimen jars, and sent them from Brooklyn to Manhattan for analysis in Gettler's laboratory. Until those results came in, investigators could "not determine what caused the death of the couple."

But, truth to tell, they rather hoped it was something else, something less ugly than cyanide.

Cyanides possess a uniquely long, dark history, probably because they grow so bountifully around us.

They flavor the leaves of the yew tree, the flowers of the cherry laurel, the kernels of peach and apricot pits, and the fat pale crunch of bitter almonds. They ooze in secretions of insects like millipedes, weave a toxic thread through cyanobacteria, massed in the floating blue-green algae along the edges of the murkier ponds and lakes, and live in plants threaded through forests and fields.

Humans recognized early the murderous potential of cyanide-rich plants. Scholars have found references to "death by peach" in Egyptian hieroglyphics, leading them to believe that those long-ago dynasties carried out cyanide executions, perhaps by making a potion from poisonous fruit pits. Centuries later cyanide became more readily available in large and lethal quantities. That happened, in part, due to some experiments by a German painter who in 1704 was only trying to improve the colors on his palette.

The artist, one Heinrich Diesbach, was a born experimenter. He spent hours in the laboratory of a Berlin chemist, trying to create a new shade of red paint. He swirled together wilder and wilder mixtures, eventually mixing dried blood, potash (potassium carbonate), and green vitriol (iron sulfate), then stewing them over an open flame. He expected the flask to yield a bloody crimson, but instead a different brilliance appeared — the deep violet-blue glow of a fading twilight. Diesbach called the vivid pigment Berlin blue; English chemists would later rename it Prussian blue.

Almost eighty years later a Swedish chemist mixed Prussian blue with an acid solution, heated the witchy, foaming result, and produced a colorless gas, undetectable but for a faint smell of bitter almonds. The gas easily condensed into a clear liquid that, even diluted with water, was an exceptionally potent acid. That corrosive liquid became popularly known as Prussic acid, although scientists preferred to call it hydrocyanic acid (from the Greek words *hydro* for water and *kyanos* for blue).

The gas was hydrogen cyanide (HCN), a deceptively simple, spectacularly lethal bundle of hydrogen, carbon, and nitrogen atoms. It could be chemically treated to produce powdery white poisonous salts, usually potassium cyanide (KCN) or sodium cyanide (NaCN). As a group, the three cyanides quickly showed themselves valuable in industrial products. Hydrogen cyanide was used in pesticides, explosives, engraving, and tempering steel, as a disinfecting agent, in creating colorful dyes, and even in making nylon. Sodium cyanide became a favored tool of the mining industry, used to etch away useless rock and extract the gold contained inside. Potassium cyanide was also used in mining, as well as in photography, electroplating, and metal polishing.

Alexander Gettler, tracking cyanide problems in New York, kept a list of accidental poisonings, such as those caused when someone with an open cut on a hand polished the family silver. The exposure was low enough that most people, after becoming miserably sick, survived. But Gettler had logged one fatality, following a meal served by a cook who failed to thoroughly wash out a pot after polishing it to a gleam inside and out. Gettler worried — no, he knew — that people using cyanides didn't appreciate how dangerous they were: "It is of considerable practical significance that hydrocyanic acid is a poison for all members of the animal kingdom."

In other words, cyanides were useful, plentiful, easy to acquire — and astonishingly lethal.

Still, most murderers tended to avoid cyanide — the poison left a too-obvious trail of evidence. The resulting corpse would be a textbook study in violent death, marked by bruising discoloration, twisted by the last convulsions, often eerily scented with cyanide's characteristic warning perfume, a faint, fruity scent of almonds. (Researchers would later find that a fair number of people carry a genetic mutation that keeps them from smelling cyanide.)

It was more popular as a suicide choice due to its reputation for acting quickly. As Gettler wrote, "The symptoms of acute poisoning proceed with almost lightning-like rapidity. Within two to five minutes after ingestion of the poison, the individual collapses, frequently with a loud scream (death scream)." In lesser amounts the poison kills more slowly, if faster than most other toxic substances. The average survival after swallowing cyanide is between fifteen and forty-five minutes. Fast or slow, it is never a kind ending. The last minutes of a cyanide death are brutal, marked by convulsions, a desperate gasping for air, a rising bloody froth of vomit and saliva, and finally a blessed release into unconsciousness.

Whether swallowed or inhaled, all members of the cyanide family kill in the same way — they shut down the body's ability to carry or absorb oxygen. In the late 1890s one daring physician swallowed a light dose of potassium cyanide to test its effects. In Gettler's day medical papers still cited his gasping cries that he was suffocating. Although the doctor survived, no one had repeated that experiment.

Cyanide's action is murderously precise. It attaches with stunning speed to protein molecules in the blood — called hemoglobins — that carry oxygen throughout the body. The poison is quicker at forming the attachment than oxygen and it binds more tightly to the hemoglobin. The blood is so tightly bound up with cyanide that the body is starved of oxygen. Cellular respiration suffers an instant "paralysis," as Gettler once put it, and the body begins to die. Enzyme production is stymied, electrical signals falter, and as muscle cells and nerve cells explosively fail, body-rattling convulsions frequently result.

After death, the bluish tones of oxygen

deprivation mottle the skin. On autopsy, the blood shows such a dark red that it sometimes appears purple. The veins leading from lung to heart are engorged with blood — evidence of the heart's desperate efforts to circulate more and more blood as the body seeks desperately for any stray trace of oxygen. In Gettler's time, the easily available cyanide salts provided further specific evidence of the poison because they were so corrosive. If swallowed, they burned their way down. An autopsy of a cyanide victim found the mucous membranes of the lips, mouth, and esophagus darkened to a bloody, ragged red — especially if the poison had been taken without food to buffer the impact. The stomach became swollen, discolored, clotted with swampy, streaky mucus produced as the cyanide salts broke down.

In the four years since Gettler had become city toxicologist, he'd investigated seventy-nine cyanide deaths, scattered across the boroughs. Forty-nine had been suicides, usually by sodium cyanide. Sodium cyanide was the cheapest form of the poison and, as research would show, was more efficient than potassium cyanide. (Sodium atoms are much smaller than potassium atoms, making room for a larger proportion of cyanide in the compound.) Most of the other deaths Gettler reviewed were accidental. Hydrogen cyanide gas was routinely used to fumigate buildings or disinfect ships. Occasionally workers were killed by the gas, especially if they returned before it had cleared.

Investigators wondered about fumigation as they looked into the deaths of Fremont and Annie Jackson at the Hotel Margaret. But the manager assured them that no fume-producing activities had occurred in the critical time period. So if indeed cyanide had killed the Jacksons, they had to have swallowed it, which was why the stomachs had been so carefully removed for chemical testing.

Gettler expected to find the usual wreckage left by the poison: the bloody, corrosive trail of cyanide through the digestive system. But it wasn't there. The tissues from the dead couple were slightly decayed but basically healthy. Still, every toxicologist knew that people reacted differently to poisons, that any known rule of evidence had the occasional exception.

So he set about doing the finer chemical tests for the poison. His plan was to check the contents of the stomachs and the tissues of the stomach muscle separately. Cyanide in the stomach would indicate only that a person had swallowed the poison. Cyanide in the stomach walls would be evidence that it had been absorbed and might even reveal how much had entered the body.

Gettler's detailed notes explained the procedure step by step. He stored the still-full stomachs in an icebox until he was ready to run his tests. He then removed the contents and separated them from the muscle tissue. From each stomach he took a healthy chunk of about 200 grams (some seven ounces) of muscle and minced it into a pinkish-gray paste. He then drained off the stomach contents into two liter-size flasks; he placed the tissue slush in two other flasks. He then dripped acid into the flasks, just a little, but enough to further break down the contents. He distilled the liquid in a steam bath and condensed it into another flask packed around with ice.

Any cyanide would be concentrated in the clear fluid contained by that last well-chilled flask.

One reliable way to then check for cyanide was called the Prussian blue test. To begin it, Gettler took a little of the distilled liquid, added some iron-rich salts, and heated the mixture. As it cooled, a muddy brown layer settled at the bottom of the flask. He then added hydrochloric acid, drop by drop, until the dirty sludge started to dissolve. If the sludge contained a high level of cyanide, a brilliant blue layer would almost immediately form in the flask. If there was only a trace of poison, there would be no blue flash. Instead the sediment would glint green before slowly turning blue.

Gettler ran the Prussian blue test on both the stomach tissue and the contents. He ran six other tests. No blue; no anything. They were all negative for cyanide. That meant the investigation was back where it had started, with two dead bodies and no good answers.

The Jackson case had all the appearance of one of those locked-room mysteries that writers of crime fiction like so much and that working detectives despise. In fact, the door to the Jacksons' apartment had been locked; a maid had found the bodies when she opened it with a hotel key in order to clean the room.

But perhaps they'd missed some clue to a clever murder. The New York State court system alone offered plenty of examples, from other cases, of the creative ways killers tried to sneak poison into their victims' food and drink.

In the previous few years alone, a Westchester man, irritated one evening because his wife wouldn't fetch his cigarettes, had placed a box of poisoned candy on the sitting room table and waited for her to sample it. A fired Mayville county clerk had sent a box of homemade candy laced with cyanide to the woman who had replaced her. A White Plains woman, irritated by the neighbor's barking dog, had substituted a bottle of milk containing cyanide for one that the milkman had delivered. A newly married woman in Olean hadn't wanted a stepson so she'd sent the six-year-old boy a box of poisoned chocolates while he was vacationing in Missouri, nearly killing the child's aunt, who ate a piece when her nephew shared his candy.

One of the most famous cyanide-by-mail murder cases in the United States had occurred in New York City at the turn of the twentieth century. It involved cyanide, had the son of a Civil War hero as the suspected murderer, and featured the city's exclusive Knickerbocker Athletic Club as the backdrop to the crime.

Shortly before Christmas 1898, the club's athletic director, Harry Cornish, received an unexpected package at home. It contained a nice little gift: a blue Tiffany box containing a bottle of Bromo-Seltzer inside a chased silver bottle holder. Cornish shared a house, owned by his aunt, with several other family members. A couple days after the holiday, his aunt developed a severe headache. Remembering the medicine he'd received in the mail, he mixed up a glass to relieve her pain. His aunt swallowed the tonic and then, to his horrified shock, collapsed to the floor, gasping for air, her face darkening to blue as she died.

Panicked family members called the doctor, who immediately detected the characteristic bitter almond smell in the medicine bottle. The resulting autopsy showed classic signs of cyanide poisoning. Anonymous poisonings by mail were usually hard to solve, but the investigators caught a break: Cornish had saved the wrapping that contained the package. A secretary at the Knickerbocker Club recognized the handwriting on the label. That led police directly to a disgruntled former club member named Roland Molineux, who had quit the club after quarreling with Cornish.

The thirty-one-year-old Molineux seemed an unlikely suspect. He was the elegant and well-educated son of a famous Civil War hero. Former Union Major General Leslie Molineux had fought in some of the war's most critical missions, supporting Grant at Richmond and Sherman during his march through Georgia. The general was so well respected and so well liked that his reputation cast a warm and protective aura around his son. At first the police found the very notion that Roland Molineux was a killer ridiculous. But mounting circumstantial evidence changed their minds.

Molineux had an account at Tiffany & Co. and had made a purchase at the Fifth Avenue store in December, which would have provided him with the familiar blue box. He worked for a family dye company, had studied chemistry, and had a personal laboratory equipped with an array of poisons used in dyes — mercury, arsenic, and cyanide-rich Prussian blue. His office was located within blocks of the post office from which the package had been mailed. And the son was nothing like his father: he was instead a man with an outsize sense of superiority. His quarrels with Cornish had involved the other's refusal to expel "lesser" families from events. He'd written to the club asking for Cornish's removal, describing him as a "vile, bad man."

The police investigation turned up something even more disturbing. A month earlier, in November 1898, another member of the

Knickerbocker Club had died unexpectedly. The dead man, Henry Barnet, had been pursuing a rather beautiful young woman whom Molineux wanted to marry. Barnet's death had been considered a natural one; the death certificate blamed a sudden weakness of the heart. But now detectives discovered that Barnet had also received an anonymous package of medicine in the mail and died shortly after taking it. They exhumed Barnet's body and discovered that the stomach and other organs contained a high concentration of cyanide.

Less than three weeks after Barnet's death, Molineux had married the woman in question. The police were sure that Molineux had killed both people, but prosecutors decided to try him only for the death of Cornish's aunt, where the evidence — including the handwriting sample — was stronger. The case went to trial in late 1899, and at its conclusion Roland Molineux was sent to Sing Sing to await execution.

But the prosecutor had made an unfortunate decision in his closing argument: he'd repeatedly talked to the jury of Barnet's death, even though Molineux had not been charged in that case. He dramatically told the jurors that he could hear not one but two voices in the night calling to him for justice: Cornish's tragically dead aunt, and Henry Barnet, "in the vigor of his youth and manhood, stricken down in that same manner . . . And will a jury of my countrymen quail before the honest and just verdict? I think not."

Molineux remained in prison almost two years, writing a book about his experiences called *The Room with the Little Door* while his father fought to clear him. He was still writing it on October 15, 1901, when the New York State Court of Appeals ruled unanimously that the references to Barnet's death had been improper and reversed the conviction. A year later the district attorney insisted on trying Roland Molineux again, convinced of his guilt. But this time the general hired an array of handwriting experts to contradict the damaging evidence of the mailing label.

Roland Molineux was acquitted in the second trial, which took place in 1902. His wife promptly divorced him. The verdict in New York drawing rooms was that the son was guilty of both cyanide poisonings but that the second jury had exonerated the father. After his acquittal, Roland Molineux remained obsessed with the life and plight of the unjustly convicted man. He wrote several more books and collaborated on a play about the criminal's plight, then suffered a mental breakdown and was committed to the New York State Hospital for the Insane in 1913. He died in the asylum four years later, at the age of fifty-one.

People who followed poison cases saw in Molineux's the same lessons as in the Rice case, or even in Mors's. Despite a clear motive and strong evidence that the victims had died of cyanide poisoning, Roland Molineux had escaped conviction. The lessons were hard to miss: poisoners were hard to catch and even harder to convict.

Meanwhile, more than a week after the bodies had been discovered, the Jackson case remained a complete mystery.

The medical examiner's office had ruled out food poisoning, due to the stiff and cold condition of the two bodies when found. In ptomaine cases, the bacterial infection tends to raise body temperature, enough that corpses retain heat longer than those killed by other means. The Jacksons' bodies had been too cold too soon to be caused by ptomaine.

Gettler had conducted a careful analysis of the couple's brain tissue for alcohol and found traces in both of them. Perhaps, the police proposed, the Jacksons had sipped some disastrous wood alcohol cocktails with their dinner. But everyone who had known the victims dismissed the idea: the Jacksons were ardent churchgoers and Prohibition supporters, they said.

The investigators greeted these denials with skepticism. Plenty of respectable people — including the mayor himself — were regulars at the speakeasies. So were many of the federal agents employed to enforce the law; dry agents were routinely hospitalized, most recently in San Francisco and Boston, after guzzling too much wood alcohol. These self-professed teetotalers had probably been sneaking a few Gin Fizzes on the side, like just about everyone else.

It was a reasonable conclusion to a case with no answers, the detectives thought. Certainly there was enough lethal liquor out there to kill every resident of the Hotel Margaret, and more.

In an interview with New York newspapers, federal Prohibition officer Izzy Einstein — the city's "champion hooch hunter," as he called himself — warned that the speakeasies were serving "the vilest concoctions masquerading as liquors that I have ever seen. I do believe a good-sized drink of this stuff would knock out the average man, even a Prohibition agent."

Einstein, a former postal clerk, and his partner, a retired cigar-store owner named Moe Smith, had signed up as Prohibition agents in the first year of the new law and refined their techniques ever since. They relied on a simple method to collect evidence for a prosecution. They would order a drink and pour a sample of it into a funnel, hidden in a vest pocket, that emptied into a small bottle. After carefully stoppering the bottle, Einstein and Smith would whip out their badges and arrest everyone involved in serving them that drink.

The duo were endlessly inventive in procuring illegal offerings. Smith had once jumped into icy water so that Einstein could rush him into a bar and beg a drink for a freezing man. They then busted the bar. They had posed as football players (when arresting an ice cream vendor who sold gin out of his cart), Texas Rangers, a Yiddish couple (Smith playing the wife), streetcar conductors, gravediggers, fishermen, and ice men. Einstein — who had a booming baritone — once introduced himself as an opera singer and gave a rousing performance in a speakeasy before closing it down.

As Einstein assured the reporters, he and his partner were far too savvy to drink the toxic liquorlike substances currently circulating. Their work, he asserted, had led them to develop "a highly developed sense of smell as regards the aroma of anything intoxicating . . . Of course, these bootleggers are getting cleverer every day and occasionally we run across a concoction that is almost odorless. Then we barely moisten our tongues to determine whether or not it has a kick. Such a test is easy to the trained hooch hunter."

Even if city agents did occasionally "enjoy a little nip now and then," he added, they indulged only in the really good liquor they'd confiscated, the "choice article." But Einstein wasn't sure that he trusted even that. For himself, he left the evidence in the stoppered bottle: "I'd rather save my stomach."

But in the Jackson case, the city's ready supply of poisonous liquor turned out not to be culpable. The deaths at the Hotel Margaret continued to drive the medical examiner and police crazy.

Gettler ran tests on the contents of every bottle, box, and container in the apartment. One of them — a sleeping tonic — had included a legal amount of ethyl alcohol. It was easily enough to account for the trace alcohol in the brain tissue but was definitely not enough to kill a person. And ethyl alcohol wasn't that poisonous anyway, Gettler noted, compared to (methyl) alcohol. He found nothing to indicate fatal alcohol poisoning.

Exasperated, one tenacious Brooklyn detective went back to the Hotel Margaret and reinterviewed every staff member he could bully into talking. This time a frightened maidservant told him something new. On the day of the Jacksons' death the basement rooms under their apartment had been sealed with paper pasted over the doors and windows. This was standard procedure when fumigators were at work. Armed with that information he soon discovered that the hotel management had been hiding the fact that the basement had been fumigated at the time when the couple had died.

Had the fumigator used hydrogen cyanide, a fairly routine procedure, for the disinfection? Water and steam pipes connected the basement to the Jacksons' rooms; could the gas have traveled up the pipes? Hydrogen cyanide was notoriously lethal, even in ridiculously small measures. If it was distilled into a liquid, a mere drop, a raindrop-sized dose (about 50 milligrams), could be fatal. During the previous summer U.S.

public health workers had accidentally killed four sailors, on two different foreign vessels, by fumigating against possible plague-carrying rats. In the second case, the steamer *Mincio,* docked at Brooklyn's Italian-American pier, had been aired out for a day before seamen returned. Still, unexpected pockets of hydrogen cyanide lingered and killed three of the crew.

Now finally the police had a real theory, one that seemed to work: the Jacksons had been overcome by cyanide gas, seeping up from the basement. Mrs. Jackson had collapsed first, falling as she staggered into the bathroom. Her husband, coming to help her, had died in the bathroom doorway. It was a good theory — except for the lack of evidence of cyanide in the bodies.

So the detectives went back to Gettler, who told them that the analysis of the stomach was useless if cyanide gas had been inhaled. He would need to take a look at the lungs to find out what they needed to know. It was a point that Gettler would emphasize when he trained young chemists. To solve a cyanide killing, they had to be very clear on how the poison was administered: "In cases of poisoning by inhalation, usually none, or only the faintest trace [of cyanide] is found in the stomach contents.

This is of tremendous importance from the medico-legal aspect."

Served with that information, the district attorney persuaded the family to let his men dig up Fremont Jackson from his burial site in Springfield, New Jersey. They removed the lungs, then reburied the corpse. The jars of grayish, somewhat slimy tissue — it *had* been more than two weeks since Jackson died — were hurried over to Gettler's Bellevue laboratory.

When the lungs were cut open, the telltale signs of cyanide poisoning paraded before them. The lining, the mucous membranes, were swollen and splattered with bloody bursts of hemorrhages, explosions of dying blood cells. And when the neat tissue slices were put through the same chemical tests that Gettler had tried with the stomach, they glowed with the eerie, evening-sky light of Prussian blue.

"In recent years, suicidal, accidental and industrial cyanide poisonings have occurred with increasing frequency," Gettler wrote in the *American Journal of Clinical Pathology*. Suicides and accidental deaths by cyanide fumigation accounted for the worst of them. By the year of the Jackson case, he'd investigated almost eighty cyanide deaths in New

York City.

In 1922, including the Jacksons, cyanide fatalities totaled four accidental deaths and ten suicides. (Starting in 1929, the suicide numbers would be higher, due to the financial catastrophes of the Depression: in 1929, 22 self-terminations by cyanide; in 1930, 34 such deaths. In 1933, according to Gettler's records, there were 49 suicides by cyanide.) But by the end of the decade fumigation deaths would virtually disappear. That was largely because the Jackson case would push Norris and Gettler to relentlessly crusade against the use of that superpoison in routine home and business fumigations. Within a few years the two of them had argued, lobbied, and embarrassed city regulators into putting an end to cyanide fumigation.

They had many reasons — aside from the obvious wish to prevent other such deaths — to avoid a repeat of the Hotel Margaret scenario.

Once Gettler found evidence of cyanide poisoning in Fremont Jackson's lungs, the medical examiner's office decided to further test the new theory of the deaths. They wanted to be sure that the cyanide could have come from fumes seeping up from the basement. Half a dozen white rats were let loose in the Jacksons' rooms, and cyanide gas was released in the basement below. In less than three hours, all the rats were dead. "The couple probably succumbed before they realized what had happened to them," Norris's office reported.

Norris and John Ruston, the district attorney in Brooklyn, were furious at the deception. They called a meeting to share their sense of outrage. The hotel manager had lied — denying any fumigation — and had simply shrugged, when reinterviewed, saying the fumigation had slipped his mind. The fumigator, for his part, had hidden in cowardly invisibility and was still not returning phone calls.

These culprits had covered up the real cause of death and sent law enforcement officials into almost two weeks of embarrassing and costly attempts to figure out what had killed a well-liked couple. If the manager and fumigator had been honest, Ruston said, he would have treated the deaths as a terrible mistake — certainly he wouldn't have brought charges. But now he wanted them punished. Ruston decided to charge them both — the fumigator, Albert Bradicich, and the manager, Eli Dupuy — with manslaughter.

If the case had justified more severe charges, he would have brought those as well.

The resulting trial was another painful lesson in the realities of poison prosecutions. The lawyers hired by Bradicich and Dupuy didn't bother to deny that the building had been fumigated on the day of the Jacksons' deaths. They didn't deny either that their clients might not have cooperated fully with the police, as they put it. The defense argument focused elsewhere: the science was no good; the Jacksons' deaths were still a mystery; the medical examiner's office had failed to prove that cyanide was responsible. Their paid experts assured them that Dr. Gettler had gotten the whole thing wrong.

The defense position was that cyanide could not be detected in a decaying body; the poison simply broke down too quickly. So the results from Jackson's lung were in error. Gettler argued back that they were misstating the medical facts. Yes, cyanide broke down, but it was not as transient as they said. The defense lawyers merely laughed — the city chemist was just trying to cover his mistakes. Bradicich's attorney based his case on the notion that Alexander Gettler was a thoroughly incompetent scientist who had missed the answer in the first analysis and faked it in the second.

To Norris's dismay, the assistant district attorney who prosecuted the case allowed his good chemist to be filleted in public. It was hard to believe, Norris raged to the prosecutor's office, that the defendants' lawyer "should have made such inexcusable statements against the character of Dr. Gettler. It is really almost unbelievable that such a thing could be done in open court without protest."

Further, Norris added, Bradicich's so-called experts had flat-out lied in court. One defense witness had claimed to have conducted a cyanide analysis on body parts obtained from the city morgue. He hadn't, and Norris could prove it: "We have been looking up at the morgue in Manhattan for the disappearance of a lung or lungs which one of the experts said he obtained for his experiments . . . No one knows anything about it and we are extremely careful about giving organs to people we do not know. I would like to see some of these medical experts punished for their nefarious testimony."

The defense lawyer had also mocked the prosecution for overreaching, trying to "build up a case by inference and make a

Roman holiday of it." He'd urged the jury to acquit on the basis of reasonable doubt of guilt and total doubt of the evidence. The tactic worked. Both defendants were acquitted on all charges.

The assistant district attorney, Joe Gallagher, explained to Gettler and Norris that toxicology was such a new science, it was awfully hard to educate and convince a jury simultaneously. He thought Gettler had done an outstanding job in the circumstances, he wrote, and thanked him for his cooperation and help. But he hoped that they understood why the case had been lost.

"I understand the situation as you describe it perfectly," Norris wrote back. "Dr. Gettler never thought the case could be put across, largely for the reasons you give in your letter. I, however, had a rather optimistic view before the end of the trial. However, I was wrong."

He sounded resigned, but in truth he wasn't. Neither was Gettler. Not at all.

In their different ways, both Norris and Gettler took the Bradicich trial personally. A few months later, Norris started a crusade to "improve the medico-legal situation," not only in New York but across the country. He was determined that the profession would gain the credibility and respect it deserved — in court and out of it.

That September Norris caught a train to Washington, D.C., to meet with representatives from other cities — a coroner's physician from Chicago, a pathologist from Johns Hopkins, a chemistry expert from Cornell Medical College, and the revered medical examiner from Boston, George McGrath, who had created one of the first professional programs in the country. They agreed to form a committee, pool their resources, and hire someone to investigate the state of forensic medicine through the country — "the training and qualifications of the men performing this important work in the various large cities" — so that they could start setting some national standards.

The Bradicich case wasn't the first in which the defense won by personally attacking a forensic scientist. That was partly because disreputable coroners' operations had tarnished the profession. Old and shoddy practices had to change, and the public had to be educated, the scientists agreed. Norris persuaded the Rockefeller Foundation to provide a small grant for their program. As he wrote to the foundation, "The most effective way to bring this matter to the public would be to contrast the European system with this country: in the former where this work as a whole is performed only by trained investigators, whereas in this country it is performed mostly by those who have no technical or practical experience."

He was proud that his office was trying to rectify that situation. But the general public perception of forensic experts undermined what he wanted to accomplish. And that, Norris wrote in a blast of anger, had gone on too long. If others didn't want to spend time changing the situation, he would do it himself.

Gettler also responded to the Bradicich trial like a man with a mission. If he'd spent late nights in the laboratory before, well, now he made them later. If by extra time and pure furious drive he could make his science more credible, he was prepared to do that.

Over the next decade and more, he would pursue cyanide studies in his laboratory and create a meticulous series of reports analyzing cyanide deaths. A 1938 paper, "The Toxicology of Cyanide," summarized his findings best and would be cited long after his death, referenced by toxicologists and government agencies into the twenty-first century.

The cyanide paper provided a chronicle of his obsession: tests with steam and with ice, chemical reactions producing brilliant yellows, sunset reds, the purplish-gray of storm clouds, the translucent green of tourmaline, kingly blues, and murky browns; bloody experiments with human organs put through a meat grinder; and grisly experiments with dogs. Every detail was carefully noted for future use.

Gettler learned that if he chilled his meat grinder in cracked ice before using it to mince the tissues, he lost less of the cyanide to heat effects. He learned that of eight standard tests for detecting cyanide in tissues, five were imprecise. He learned that steadily adding iron compounds and hydrochloric acid to his minced tissue was reliable, every time resulting in the giveaway blue of cyanide. He tried different tests, seeking the smallest trace of detectable cyanide. He ran eight additional tests trying, eventually successfully, to tease out one part per million. He used those tests to find out whether the human body naturally harbored a baseline level of cyanide. To do that, he analyzed hundreds of livers and brains, lungs and kidneys, from people who had died of other causes. In people who had never been exposed to the poison, he found no trace of natural cyanide, leading him to conclude, "either that no cyanide whatever is present in normal tissue distillates, or that the minute quantity of cyanide that may be present lies below the sensitivity of the test."

He spent time figuring out the precise routes that cyanide took in the body, at one point using four dogs to compare the effects of inhaling the poison versus ingesting it. No one would describe these experiments as pretty, but he justified them as pure necessity. Two dogs received measured doses of potassium cyanide through a stomach tube; the others were forced to inhale hydrogen cyanide. The latter two animals were strapped to an operating table with their jaws taped shut. A cone-shaped mask would be placed over a dog's nose and mouth, taped in place, and sealed with Vaseline to make it airtight. Once the mask was fixed, hydrogen cyanide gas would be piped into the cone until the dog died.

The results provided some of the first measured evidence of how quickly cyanide kills, dispelling the myth that victims neatly drop dead on the spot. When Gettler gave a dog 50 milligrams of cyanide (a little less than 2 ounces), the animal died in 21 minutes. When he cut the dose to 20 milligrams, the dog lived for 2 hours and 35 minutes. When inhaled, less of the poison was needed to kill, and it worked more quickly, but again not instantly. One gassed dog, for instance, breathed in about 10 milligrams of cyanide; he was dead in 15 minutes.

The animal studies — later confirmed in analyses of human cyanide victims — showed that the poison is absorbed differently depending on how it is taken. When it is inhaled, it blows through the body, concentrates in the lungs, and swims through the bloodstream into the brain, the heart, and the liver. When swallowed, the poison is absorbed much more slowly. Necropsies (or animal autopsies) of the two dogs that were fed cyanide found that much of the poison, between 38 and 83 percent, was still in the stomach when they died, which helped explain why they died more slowly than the dogs that had breathed in the poison.

Remembering the Jackson case, Gettler made a point of exploring what happened to cyanide in a decaying body. He took slices of livers and brains and lungs from the bodies of cyanide victims, noting the poison content of each. He placed those pieces of tissue into containers and then left them to rot on a shelf in his laboratory. He checked the results at one week, two weeks, three weeks, and four, looking far beyond the time that Fremont Jackson had been buried so that he could be absolutely sure of the conclusion.

"During this time putrefaction developed to a high degree," he wrote with serious understatement concerning those month-old organ slices. He analyzed the decaying tissues for cyanide and compared the amount to the levels he'd measured when they were still fresh. He found that decomposition altered the poison readings by the barest amount. Even after four weeks, 90 percent of the original poison content could still be detected, once again validating his testimony in the 1922 case.

Gettler investigated another contention made in the Bradicich case, that even if cyanide was present in the old man's body, it was meaningless. The defense experts had insisted that the body naturally produced its own cyanide as a part of decomposition. He was determined to set that straight as well. So he took samples from eight different organs, all taken from bodies of people who had died natural deaths, and sealed them in glass flasks. Every week for the following two months, he removed one for analysis.

During the first week, decay produced

trace amounts of cyanide — about 0.03 milligrams per 100 grams of tissue — but after that the poison seemed to disintegrate. By the end of two months, cyanide could not be detected at all. At its strongest, though, it was a mere whisper, a fading breath in the test tube, nothing close to the levels he'd found in Fremont Jackson. "Putrefaction therefore should in no way interfere with deciding a cyanide poisoning case," he concluded.

It had taken him years in a laboratory, silent with the emptiness of night hours, to get his answer to the Jackson case. If Gettler could have carried his findings back in time to that courtroom, he would have done so and perhaps changed the outcome. He found satisfaction instead in building a better science out of an unhappy episode. Next time, he promised himself, such legal sabotage would not succeed.

Still, it might not have particularly bothered Gettler that decades later, in 1980, the Hotel Margaret, long abandoned, would undergo renovations during which it accidentally burned to the ground. No one in Charles Norris's office held fond memories of that shining ornament of a building. Those coppery roofs and elegant balconies, those devious employees and that seeping

poisonous gas; all of it reminded them only
of mistakes that they intended not to make
again.

# FOUR:
## ARSENIC (As)
### 1922–1923

The weather in that summer of 1922 held steady at what the newspapers like to call "fair," the skies a gas-flame blue, the temperatures hovering near 80 degrees. On the last day of July, as Lillian Goetz's mother would forever recall, the morning was another warm one. She offered to make seventeen-year-old Lillian a box lunch, but the girl refused. It was too hot to eat much; she'd just grab a quick sandwich at a lunch counter, she said.

Lillian worked as a stenographer in a dress goods firm occupying a small set of offices in the Townsend Building, at the bustling corner of 25th and Broadway. There were plenty of quick eateries nearby, tucked among the offices and shops and small hotels. Lillian, like many of her co-workers, often stepped over to the Shelbourne Restaurant and Bakery, just half a block south on Broadway.

The Shelbourne catered to the office trade, opening in the morning, closing in the early afternoon. Stenographers and secretaries in their bright summer hats and stylish short skirts, businessmen and office managers in their dark tailored suits, crowded daily along its wooden counters and small square tables, hurrying through a meal of hot soup with fresh-baked rolls, a sandwich, coffee, and a slice of the bakery's renowned peach cake or berry pie.

According to police reports, on July 31 Lillian ordered a tongue sandwich, coffee, and a slice of huckleberry pie. It was the pie that killed her.

By early afternoon sixty people had been rushed to nearby hospitals after eating lunch at the Shelbourne, and by the end of the day, six of them, including Lillian Goetz, were dead. The scream of ambulances on lower Broadway was so constant that a number of people called the police in a panic, fearing that the whole city had caught fire.

The Townsend Building, where Goetz worked, was an 1896 neoclassical structure that normally conveyed a stately limestone sense of calm. Now it served as backdrop to a scene of hysteria. Office workers collapsed on every one of the twelve floors, convulsing, vomiting, gasping in misery. Doctors armed with stomach pumps — at least ten pumps were put to use throughout the building — hurried from floor to floor, crisis to crisis. In the excited words of the city newspapers, "Panic prevailed on some floors in the Townsend building as one employee after another turned pale, and then blue and began to complain of intense pain."

Gradually the doctors began comparing symptoms, notes, and stories. It led them to realize two things: that every victim had lunched at the Shelbourne Restaurant, and that almost all had eaten either blackberry or huckleberry pie for dessert. The physicians called the health department and the medical examiner's office to report their suspicions.

The following day Charles Norris and Frank Monaghan, the acting health commissioner, made a joint announcement. Arsenic had been found in the piecrusts and rolls served at the Shelbourne. Additional tests showed that none of the ingredients — flour, butter, salt — stored at the restaurant contained any poison. Therefore the investigators suspected that the arsenic had been added to the dough after it was mixed, perhaps into the covered dough bowl stored in the kitchen refrigerator.

In other words, Norris and Monaghan agreed, this was not a matter of a kitchen accident, a baker using flour from grain tainted by an arsenic pesticide. Someone had planned this: "the food had been poisoned with malicious intent."

Knowing the poison is never the same as knowing the killer. The police wished it were. They had no answer as to who might have done this. No answer as to why anyone would wish to harm a seventeen-year-old stenographer, working to help out her family, whose mother repeatedly told police that she only, only wished she had made that box lunch.

The previous October, in an unnervingly similar incident, two lunch patrons had been killed by arsenic at a restaurant down in the financial district. At that little eatery, near the old Liberty Street post office, health inspectors had at first suspected food poisoning. But then Alexander Gettler had isolated lethal amounts of poison in both men's bodies.

The police had not identified a suspect in the killings at the Postal Lunch eatery, had never even come close. Maybe that was why people quit going to the eatery, which was now closed down. One of the first fears expressed by the police department was that the same poisoner had now moved up to Broadway; that this killer just enjoyed causing death, someone — detectives speculated — like the still-infamous Jean Crones.

Years earlier Crones had worked as an assistant chef at the exclusive University Club in downtown Chicago. In his spare time he belonged to the city's thriving community of anarchists, an outspoken opponent of what he considered the government oppression ruining the country. But his political views never explained — neither to his kitchen colleagues nor to his political allies — why on February 10, 1916, while making sauces for a dinner honoring Catholic bishops, he added a liberal seasoning of arsenic to the meat stock.

Seventy-five of the three hundred people at the dinner became rapidly, horribly sick. In the ensuing maelstrom of shouting emergency workers and terrified diners, Crones simply walked out of the club and caught a train to the East Coast. He was never apprehended, although he briefly stopped in New York to mail police-baiting letters to the Manhattan newspapers. His mocking notes suggested that the incompetent Chicago police should take lessons in detection, perhaps enrolling in a correspondence school, although he doubted they would since "the city of Chicago officials are fools."

Investigators came to believe that Crones had simply stirred in poison as an experiment, for the pure pleasure of seeing the results. They hoped that this wasn't true of their New York poisoner, who seemed more adept than Crones. The Chicago chef had loaded far too much arsenic into the soup, causing many people to put down their spoons at the metallic taste, preventing them from falling ill. Those who kept eating became sick quickly, but doctors who rushed to the scene were able to administer rapid treatment. As a result, no one had died in Crones's experiment.

At the Shelbourne, as at the Postal Lunch, the poisoner had calculated a much more effective dose, high enough to kill but low enough to fool the victims. The lunch patrons at the Broadway eatery had had time to return to work before they became ill. Their illness attracted medical attention but not quickly enough to save everyone. If the unidentified Shelbourne suspect and the never-caught Postal Lunch killer were the same person, then police were looking for a killer who knew all too well how to pick a poison, how to use it, and how to disappear.

Pure arsenic is a dark, grayish element, classed among the heavy metal poisons, often found in ores extracted from mines. It easily combines with other naturally occurring chemicals; heated with oxygen, for instance, it becomes a white, crumbly powder, the linking of two arsenic atoms with three of oxygen. In this form it is called arsenic trioxide ($As_2O_3$) or white arsenic.

White arsenic, the poison used at the Shelbourne, was a favorite of some of history's most feared poisoners, ones who made Jean Crones look like the amateur he was. At the top of the list were Lucretia and Cesare Borgia, feared in fifteenth-century Italy for their ruthless mixture of politics and poison. The Borgias used white arsenic preferentially but experimented with different ways to make it more deadly. They would cook it into a more intense solution, mixing it with other poisons. They eventually created a poison they called *la cantarella,* which according to legend was so dangerous that the formula was destroyed after their deaths.

Basic arsenic is also deadly; the first recorded case of homicide with the pure element was reported in 1740, when a girl poisoned her father and three sisters by serving them a dish of dried pears that had been boiled in water containing rocky ore from a nearby mine. But for criminal uses, white arsenic is a better tool, slipped easily into food or drink. Its usefully murderous properties explained why, centuries after the Borgias, the poison earned another nickname: the inheritance powder. One of the best-known nineteenth-century American forensic scientists, Columbia University chemistry professor Rudolph Witthaus, coauthor of the massive 1896 tome *Medical Jurisprudence, Forensic Medicine and Toxicology*, had once tried to estimate arsenic's popularity as a murder weapon. He selected 820 arsenic-caused deaths, recorded between 1752 and 1889 — and found that almost half were homicides. (The rest were split fairly evenly between accidents and suicides.)

In Europe, by Witthaus's analysis, arsenic accounted for the largest percentage of nineteenth-century criminal poisonings. In France, for example, between 1835 and 1880, arsenic was used in almost 40 percent of all poison murders. "In the United States, we are under the impression that arsenic still holds the first place in frequency of criminal administration," Witthaus wrote. But at the time of his analysis, the United

States lacked the statistical information available in France. As a rough measure, Witthaus interviewed New York State attorneys and determined that from 1879 to 1889, there had been thirty-one indictments for poison murder in twelve counties. Half of those were arsenic murders; in every case, white arsenic was specifically to blame.

A primary reason for arsenic's popularity was that when mixed into food and drink, it is extremely difficult to taste. An over-the-top dose, the kind Jean Crones had used, was different. If arsenic was swallowed in undiluted form, that was different too. Witthaus and other scientists taste-tested small amounts of pure white arsenic and found it to be rather nasty. It was hot, tasters said; it was acrid, sweetish, metallic, and rough. But when the poison was added to soup, liquor, or a cup of hot coffee, the other flavorings easily masked it. Arsenic was "under the most favorable circumstances faint" in taste, Witthaus noted. In interviews with 822 people who had survived arsenic poisoning, he reported that only fifteen thought the food had tasted in any way strange. Six talked of a bitter taste, eight complained of a metallic feeling in the mouth, and one woman said she was aware of a "nauseous" taste. Witthaus doubted the latter, noting that as the unpleasant taste "escaped the notice of 14 other persons who ate of the same poisoned pudding, it was probably more imaginary than real."

White arsenic mixes especially beautifully into alcoholic drinks, which tend to hide even a faint metallic sensation. One group of cheerful drinkers had shared a bottle of port wine and suffered from fairly severe arsenic poisoning, but "not the least taste was perceived by any of the parties." Sometimes people complained of a sandy feel in their mouths; they seemed unusually sensitive to the rough texture of the powder, even mixed into food. In an 1860 New Jersey case, a man had murdered his wife by rubbing white arsenic into an apple. During the trial he acknowledged that "she said there was something gritty on it," but she'd eaten anyway, thinking he just hadn't washed it well. Mostly, though, ground extra-fine and mixed into baked goods, as at the Shelbourne, arsenic proved an almost undetectable ingredient.

In fact, handled with skill by a calculating murderer, the poison seemed to engender a homicidal overconfidence. In 1872, one notorious British murderer, Mary Ann Cotton, killed fifteen people, including all the children of her five husbands, and several neighbors who irritated her, before she was caught in 1872, tried, and hanged. "Arsenic has also been," Witthaus wrote, "in almost every instance, the agent used by those who, having succeeded in a first attempt at secret poisoning, have seemed to develop a lust for murder and have continued to add to their list of victims until their very number has aroused suspicion and led to detection."

At the time of the Shelbourne killings, scientists were still not sure how arsenic killed; the action of cyanide was far better understood. Not for decades would molecular biologists work out the method by which arsenic targets key enzymes, disrupting metabolism within cells throughout the body, breaking the system down cell by poisoned cell. Part of the problem for early toxicology researchers was that arsenic, as one complained, is a great mimic.

Physicians often mistook symptoms of arsenic poisoning for natural diseases, especially if the victim was dosed gradually. General practitioners and emergency room doctors had misdiagnosed arsenic deaths as influenza; as cholera, which also causes severe gastrointestinal distress; and as heart disease, which also causes gasping shortness of breath. Such errors were found only when a suspicious relative who was sure the victim had been healthy, and distrusted a husband or wife, demanded an autopsy.

From the poisoner's perspective, arsenic became a risky choice when doctors looked directly at the body. With the stubborn, solid constitution of any metallic element, it breaks down extremely slowly compared to organic poisons and can be detected decades after death in a victim's hair and fingernails. Even worse for those who hope to avoid detection, arsenic tends to slow down the natural decomposition of human tissue, often creating eerily well-preserved corpses. Toxicologists refer to this effect as arsenic "mummification." Witthaus reported that one body, exhumed after fifty-four weeks in the ground, "did not differ from a living person" in appearance except for the patches of mold growing on his face. "The growth of molds is not interfered with by arsenic," he added austerely.

The other complication for the would-be poisoner was that, responding to arsenic's long history of criminal use, scientists had found numerous ways to test for it in human tissue and recognize it in an autopsy. Tests to extract arsenic from a corpse had been available for almost one hundred years and had steadily improved in the intervening period. More chemical procedures, better developed tests, and more detailed autopsy information were available for detecting arsenic than any other poison. For those studying the dead, arsenic was so easy to find that one might almost imagine it glowing in the dark, flashing its message of murder.

Charles Norris liked to get his hands bloody in the morgue on a regular basis.

A good medical examiner, he believed, kept his autopsy tools sharp and his pathology skills honed. Plus, truthfully, he was bored by a job that consisted of little besides paperwork, meeting with other government officials, and harassing the mayor. The mass murders at the Shelbourne needed to be handled by an authority figure, Norris decided.

He would do the autopsies himself.

The Bellevue autopsy room was quiet and cool, with high ceilings and white plastered walls. Lights hung brightly over each long marble dissecting table; at every table's foot was a deep rectangular copper basin with hot running water, to keep hands and instruments clean. As the standard manual reminded pathologists, blood and fluids that dried on the fingers could be "unpleasant" and dull the sensitivity needed for the operation.

The instruments lay in bristling rows. There was the section knife, with its short thick blade and heavy handle, used for making long incisions, and slim scalpels ready to make the finer cuts. At Bellevue they always laid out three instruments for probing the brain: a deep cutter, with a six-inch handle and six-inch blade "so strong it does not bend or feather too easily" to slice through the dura, the tough membrane protecting the brain; a thin, two-sided blade with a rounded tip used for incisions; and a pick, used to free the brain from the spinal cord so that it could be removed from the body.

There were delicate tissue-cutting scissors and powerful bone scissors used to crunch through cartilage and thinner bones; dissecting forceps; at least one good butcher's saw for the bigger bones; smaller saws for tasks like removing the spinal cord; brass and wooden foot-rules (twelve-inch rulers); tape measures, measuring glasses and calipers; large scales to weigh the whole body and small scales to weigh the pieces; glass-stopped jars to hold the organs for poison analysis; and the usual assortment of sponges, pails, vessels, plates, and bottles that collected in all postmortem rooms.

Before the first cut, a pathologist like Norris would need to take detailed notes on a cadaver's outward appearance. Victims of acute arsenic poisoning tended to become so violently sick that their bodies had the slightly shrunken, emaciated look of severe dehydration. Often their hands and feet looked slightly blue due to lack of circulating oxygen. If, on the other hand, the poison had been administered gradually, the victims' skin tended to turn yellow, even occasionally a kind of parchment brown, and scaly patches appeared on the hands and feet.

When it was time to begin an autopsy, the corpse was laid on its back, with its head dangling just over the edge of the table so that the neck was pushed forward. The first cut into the trunk of the body was a Y-cut with the section knife, two deep slices inward from a few inches below each shoulder to a point under the breastbone and then straight down through the abdominal muscles. (Undertakers had demanded that technique, rather than a slash straight down the center from the throat, so that clothing would easily cover the incisions during an open casket ceremony.)

Once the flaps of skin were peeled back, the sternum and a triangular section of ribs could be removed and the protective muscles sliced open, yielding access to the organs below. Like other pathologists, Norris followed a set routine. He inspected each organ and described its condition in detail. Since poison was suspected, he removed the organs, placed them in sealed glass jars, and sent them upstairs to Gettler's laboratory.

In the case of arsenic, this was indeed bloody work. The entire body had to be sliced apart. Since the early nineteenth century, scientists had known that the poison accumulated everywhere. They'd found it in the liver, spleen, kidneys, heart, lungs, brain, stomach, intestines, and even the muscle walls themselves.

White arsenic (the compound isolated from the Shelbourne's pastry) wrecked the stomach, leaving it smudged with bloody lesions; the mucous membrane lining would be swollen, yellowish, and patched with scarlet. Under a microscope, the membrane would sparkle with tiny arsenic crystals — the same ones that caused the gritty sensation in food. The poison tracked similar damage through the intestines. The heart often contained loosely formed blood clots. In a quick killing, little evidence was found in the liver and kidneys, but in a slow, chronic arsenic poisoning — favored by killers hoping to mimic the decline of a natural disease — both organs became diseased, showing signs of fatty degeneration.

It took only a day for Norris to compare his autopsy notes with Gettler's organ-by-organ chemical analyses. The results weren't really a surprise. Both of them had found the same thing — poison fanned through the bodies like a sparkling dust blown by a prevailing wind.

The police continued to hope, sincerely, that they were not hunting a stranger killer. They preferred that the motive be personal, sabotage maybe, and that the murders had been committed by someone with a grudge against the management.

They'd interviewed the Shelbourne's owner, Samuel Drexler, who was in a state of pure shouting rage. Most of his thirty-two employees were still sick. They had eaten leftover pastry, when the lunch rush finished, and had been felled along with the customers. There was no way, according to the proprietor, that the poison could have been mixed in accidentally.

The exterminator whom Drexler employed did not use arsenic-based pesticides;

the restaurant's wallpaper was not tinted with one of the well-known arsenic-dye greens. Neither did he accept a tentative police theory that one of his competitors might have crept into the kitchen and poisoned the dough to harm his business. He also rejected the idea of a crazed arsenic killer roaming the city.

"That is entirely out of the question," he snapped to reporters. "No one sneaked in." But he did accept the idea that someone bore a grudge: "This was absolutely malicious and intentional." As he told detectives, his own suspicions fell on the two bakers in his kitchen, who could easily have mixed an extra ingredient into the dough. Notably, neither of them had fallen ill on the fatal Monday.

Neither the baker nor his assistant — a teenage boy and friend of the baker — would admit to mixing up the suspect dough. Each insisted that the other had done it. "Is that so?" Drexler replied to the reporters jostling around his restaurant. "Their stories conflict, do they? Well, I am not in a position to throw any light on that." He had given the authorities plenty of information to help them solve the case, he added, but his own impression was that "they are completely baffled."

He posted a sign on the door of his closed restaurant, announcing that he would pay $1,000 for information leading to the arrest of the killer.

A major difficulty in finding the murderer was that almost anyone in New York City — or anywhere else — could acquire arsenic with little effort. Every day people walked into drugstores, grocery stores, garden supply stores and bought some version of the poison for the most practical reasons.

Arsenic was mixed into tonics like the popular Fowler's Solution, used for skin treatments, prescribed by doctors, dispensed at drugstores. It was available as a weed killer, a bug killer, and a rat killer. Hardware stores, groceries, and farm and garden supply shops offered up white arsenic in remarkable variety. There was Rough on Rats, a grayish powder made of 10 percent soot and 90 percent arsenic trioxide; Rat Dynamite, 9 percent bran and 91 percent arsenic; Lyon's Poisoned Cheese, a soft pale block containing some 93.5 percent white arsenic. William's Fly Paper, Dutcher's Fly Paper, and Daisy Fly Killer were all laced with arsenic, easily leached out simply by soaking them in water.

Arsenic was the primary ingredient in a

number of dyes that were especially popular in the nineteenth century and sold under such names as Scheele's Green, Paris Green, Emerald Green, Parrot Green, and Vienna Green. Mixing arsenic with copper and hydrogen yielded shades that ranged from the brilliant color of a new-leafed tree to the softer tones of a shaded moss. Over the years arsenic-based dyes were used to color fabric, the artificial leaves on hats and wreaths, cardboard boxes, greeting cards, labels, candles, India rubber balls, oil paint, artificial plants made of tin, Venetian blinds, carpets, soap, and faux malachite for jewelry. As the Shelbourne's proprietor had noted, arsenic-green wallpaper remained common through the city (though not in his particular restaurant). But even untainted wallpaper could be made poisonous by paperhangers who liked to mix a little arsenic into their horse-hoof paste, thinking it would help keep rats out of the walls.

At the Shelbourne, of course, the possibility of accidental arsenic contamination had been quickly dismissed. The poison had been too carefully mixed into the dough to be a mistake — exactly the reason so many suspected that the bakers were responsible. The senior baker even had something of a motive. He admitted to the police that he had heard a rumor that he was going to be fired. It had turned out to be untrue, but he had realized that his job was safe only after the mass poisoning. The homicide department assigned plainclothes detectives to shadow the bakers. Other detectives interviewed kitchen staff at nearby restaurants, hunting for gossip or evidence of simmering resentments at the Shelbourne. Beat officers were sent to canvass shops for arsenic sales.

As the investigation unfolded, restaurants around the city reported that their customers were firmly rejecting all offers of blackberry and huckleberry pie for dessert.

Poisoned pie wasn't the only murderous problem the police were grappling with that summer. Prohibition had cranked up the level of violence in the city; gunfights rattling the streets were becoming relatively routine. The business of illegal alcohol had quickly become a lucrative gift to the city's gangs, who'd built newly efficient organizations to manage the multimillion-dollar bootlegging industry.

Racketeers across the United States purchased 80 percent of the liquor distilled in Canada; they'd invested in small fleets of boats to smuggle alcohol (and Chinese immigrants) in from the Caribbean; they'd opened "import businesses" for taking undercover liquor orders and advertised their wares by placing flyers on car windshields or slipping order forms under apartment doors. They were operating stills in all corners of the city. In July federal agents Izzy Einstein and Moe Smith raided a pharmaceutical laboratory in the Bronx and found three hundred-gallon stills, seventeen barrels of industrial alcohol, and twenty-two barrels of redistilled alcohol, which they described as "rat poison."

Rat poison or not, the gangs were fighting with terrifying intensity to control its distribution.

Barely a week after the Shelbourne poisoning, bootleggers' gun battles exploded again around the city. A gunman opened fire on a gang leader walking down Second Avenue past a millinery shop; the spray of bullets killed two bodyguards and punched holes through the gangster's straw boater before he ducked into the shop, dived through the hat displays, and fled out the back door. A few days later, on August 11, a revenge hit was made on the failed assassin outside a 12th Avenue restaurant. The shooter, a rising young gangster named Lucky Luciano, killed his target, and injured an eight-year-old girl who was unfortunately nearby as well as a taxi driver waiting for a fare in his parked cab.

A depressing similarity between the gangster shootings and the Shelbourne poisonings was the absence of witnesses. People who offered evidence in gangster shootings frequently ended up dead; out of fear few came forward with information. In the poison pie case, the killers worked in successful secrecy. No one had observed the mixing of arsenic dough. No one had tracked down a poison purchase by either suspect. The police department's dogged inquiry and surveillance had failed to turn up any solid information for a prosecution.

"There is no greater mistake than to arrest a man on insufficient evidence," the Manhattan district attorney announced, conceding that they had no real suspect and no immediate hope of finding one. "We cannot now show who possessed the arsenic and we cannot produce any person with a motive which seems sufficient. All we can do is follow every possible clue. This takes time. We believe that the perpetrator of this crime will eventually be caught and punished."

But realistically, the prosecutor doubted it. The Shelbourne Restaurant killer would never go down as a famous poisoner; he would never be remembered the way Mary Ann Cotton was. But from a poisoner's perspective, he'd probably accomplished something better. Cotton was hanged, after all.

He walked away.

Only two years into the great Prohibition experiment, the State of New York was ready to give it up. Where were the high moral standards, the uplifted culture, and the return to prewar innocence promised by supporters of the Eighteenth Amendment? So far the effects seemed almost the opposite, considering the street shootings, the increasingly brazen speakeasy trade, and the mounting deaths from poisoned alcohol.

Even by federal estimates, two-thirds of the so-called "whiskey" (as described by the Treasury Department) currently sold in city drink establishments was denatured alcohol, redistilled to remove the worst of the poisons, colored a golden brown with food coloring, and completely dangerous. Twelve people had died in one month from "rum" purchased in the Red Hook neighborhood of Brooklyn. The mixture sold from the back room of a corner grocery for fifty cents a pint was undiluted wood alcohol. Even as such deaths were reported, people continued to drink — defiantly, mockingly, determinedly — until by 1922, arrests for public drunkenness in New York City had topped 11,000, compared to a mere 7,028 in the year before Prohibition took effect.

Like many states, New York had passed a law providing law enforcement support for the outlawing of alcohol. But by the time Lucky Luciano sprayed bullets across 12th Avenue, support for state policing of Prohibition had shifted into anger at the regulations and their effects. Republican Governor Nathan Miller, who had supported dry enforcement, was defeated in his 1922 bid for reelection by former governor Al Smith, an uncommonly outspoken wet Democrat. After six months of quarreling, the state legislature passed an act to repeal New York's Prohibition enforcement law. The bill went to Smith in May 1923.

Returned to the governor's office, which he had lost in 1920, Smith found himself conflicted over whether to sign the bill into law. Another powerful state Democrat, Assemblyman Franklin Delano Roosevelt, warned him to keep his ambitions in mind; Smith wanted to stay governor and hoped to run for president eventually. Roosevelt, who also opposed Prohibition, nonethless suspected that signing the bill would damage Smith's national chances. The prominent Prohibitionist publisher Frank Gannett told Smith that his newspapers would never support him again if he signed the bill. The leaders of the Anti-Saloon League predicted violent clashes, approaching a civil war, if New York undermined national policy. On the opposite side, the Democratic party machine, controlled by Tammany Hall, informed Smith that if he failed to roll back the hated dry law, he would never hold state office again.

On June 1 Smith officially put an end to New York's Prohibition legislation, trying to portray his action as a reasonable response to unreasonable pressures. He wasn't legalizing drink or neutralizing the Eighteenth Amendment, he insisted. He was just returning the responsibility for enforcing an unpopular law to the federal government, which was, after all, responsible for the whole debacle.

Even in the tidy Brooklyn home of Alexander Gettler, it was impossible to avoid the complications wrought by Prohibition. Gettler, his wife, and their seven-year-old son, Joseph, occupied the law-abiding top floor of the family home.

But only one stair-flight down was lawlessness. His in-laws who occupied the rest of the house had set up a bathroom brewery on the second floor. They were willing to heed his warnings about buying alcohol at the corner store, but they weren't willing to give up drinking it.

Gettler might be the city's chief toxicologist. His analyses of illegal alcohol might provide evidence in countless cases against owners of backroom stills and bootlegged bottles of whiskey. But he knew better than to take on his wife and the seven other Irish-Americans occupying the house.

He wasn't all that fond of Prohibition anyway; he'd analyzed the corpses of too many people felled by wood alcohol to believe that it was about saving people. So he didn't mind drinking home-brewed beer with his family. Besides, he was working hard enough to want a drink every once in a while.

Gettler was a workaholic, always, and in the summer of 1923 he was juggling three jobs: associate professor of chemistry at New York University, city toxicologist, and chemical pathologist for Bellevue and Allied Hospitals. He was beginning to earn a reputation outside the city as well.

In the spring of 1923 he'd published a how-to paper on detecting the industrial solvent benzene in cadavers. It was the first major research report on the subject in eight years (the previous one being a German paper showing that the compound could be isolated in animal organs). He had decided to tackle benzene because, as he wrote, "nothing of importance has been accomplished since then" and because its increased use in automobile garages, where it handily dissolved grease from dirty engine parts, now posed a real public health risk. Gettler's paper, published in the *Journal of Pharmacology and Experimental Therapeutics,* concerned the case of a sixteen-year-old boy found mysteriously dead on the floor of a small garage in the Bronx. The teenager had been filling cans with the solvent shortly before collapsing. But the autopsy findings had been inconclusive, except for bloody congestion in all organs.

The problem with benzene was that it was exceptionally difficult to extract from a corpse. It could be teased out in only the tiniest amounts — sometimes no more than 0.05 grams (0.001763 of an ounce). That wasn't enough poison to be caught by existing tests, which were not sensitive to such barely there amounts. So Gettler invented a different approach: he concentrated the trace amounts of benzene by running them through a series of acid solutions and then drying the mixture to a yellowish dust, which could be used to create a stronger solution. His new method found benzene in the liver, brain, blood, fat, lungs, spleen, and heart of the dead boy. As a result, the medical examiner's office issued a public warning to garage owners that they should ventilate their buildings when handling the solvent. As Gettler reported, the fumes had killed the boy in less than two hours.

Gettler's benzene work also went into a chapter on poisons that he'd written for a new textbook, *Legal Medicine and Toxicology*. The book was edited by a trio of forensic scientists, including Chicago toxicologist Walter Haines, a famously fanatical scientist who had once paid a circus glass eater to swallow ground glass so that he could see whether the tiny fragments caused serious internal damage. (They didn't.) Gettler's chapter provided detailed information on wood alcohol, formaldehyde, chloral hydrate (sometimes called knock-out drops), chloroform and ether, the cyanides, camphor, turpentine, carbolic acid, coal tar (cresol), salicylic acid (the primary ingredient in aspirin), aniline dyes, digitalis, and even poison ivy and sumac, as well as solvents like benzene.

Ever since the fiasco of the Shelbourne Restaurant case, Gettler had also worked at improving the speed and sensitivity of detecting arsenic in human tissues. That work — as well as his growing reputation as a chemical detective — would lead him into one of the most troubling cases of his career. In his spare time (partly to help pay for his son Joe's tuition at St. John's Prep in Brooklyn) Gettler took on some consulting work in other jurisdictions. Just a few weeks after New York repealed its state Prohibition rules, he was hired by the defense attorneys for a young New Jersey woman who was accused of killing family members with arsenic.

His testimony, which helped free her, would later form part of the background story of a remarkably twisted arsenic killer nicknamed "America's Lucretia Borgia" by the tabloid newspapers.

Mary Frances Creighton, Fanny to her friends, was a rather lovely twenty-four-year-old that summer of 1923. She had curling dark hair and pale skin, "deep, luminous eyes" (according to the *New York Evening Post*), and lush "petulant lips" (according to the *New York American*).

The *New York Times* more sedately described her as a "comely brunette" and "a young mother." She had a three-year-old daughter, Ruth, and an infant son, John Jr. The baby had been delivered while both she and her husband, John, were being held in jail on murder charges.

The newspapers ran few photos of the pudgy, sandy-haired husband. But Fanny Creighton willingly posed for admiring photographers in a demure long-sleeved black dress, despite the summer heat, her eyes lowered, a carved silver cross hanging at her neck, and her infant cradled in her arms.

Resembling a Madonna, she seemed the least likely person to have killed a younger brother for a mere $1,000.

John Creighton and Mary Frances Avery had been longtime friends when they'd married in 1919. He was the son of an executive with the Pennsylvania Railroad Company. She, her brother, and two sisters were orphans, cared for by affluent grandparents.

The newlyweds moved in with Creighton's parents, who owned a big two-story home in Newark's comfortable Roseville neighborhood. They shared the space for a year until 1920, when his mother died at age forty-seven of a sudden attack of ptomaine. His father, also forty-seven, died the following year, of a heart ailment.

The young couple kept to themselves, John working as a clerk, Frances caring for her daughter in the tree-shaded house on North Seventh Street. She was unfriendly, the neighbors complained, unsociable when they came to call. Perhaps, the detectives thought, she had just been lonely when she first invited her eighteen-year-old brother to visit.

Her brother, Charles Avery, and her sisters still lived nearby with their maternal grandparents. Frances did not get along with her sisters — they'd been quarreling over the inheritance from their parents — but in early 1923 her brother had come to spend a weekend.

She persuaded him to return and stay for a while, helping him find a job as a clerk in a neighborhood store; he also swept floors and stacked boxes. Several months later, in early April, the boy began suffering from ill health. He felt sick enough to visit a doctor, complaining of a dull ache in his abdomen and a perpetual thirst that dried his mouth and furred his tongue. The doctor diagnosed a mild infection and prescribed a tonic. A week later, on April 12, the boy came back. He was now constantly nauseated and had developed a burning sore throat. The doctor increased the medication, but the boy got steadily worse.

On the night of April 20 Charles Avery suffered a seizure. Frances called a neighbor and asked her to come over, saying that her brother was making a strange noise in his throat. But the woman refused; she'd been a close friend of the elder Creightons and she didn't like the new mistress of the house well enough to come help. The doctor was summoned, and to his shock, he found the boy dying, vomiting uncontrollably, his limbs stiffening and shaking.

What had he done wrong? the doctor wondered. He'd had no idea the boy was so ill. He called the county physician, asking him for advice on filling out the death certificate, recounting the whole case history over the telephone. The two doctors finally agreed that it must have been one of those rare, violent attacks of gastroenteritis — like the one that had killed Creighton's mother — and so the doctor stated on the death certificate.

And there it might have stayed — except for the anonymous letter.

■ ■ ■ ■

"Is death not ground for suspicion?" the letter writer asked the police, insisting that Avery's death was peculiar, as had been the earlier ones. "This boy feared his sister as he feared death . . . I am very sorry that I cannot sign my name. I am just an outsider who is very fond of this boy. Please act quickly and beware. You will find it hard to trap this liar."

It was enough to send the detectives out to ask a few questions of the attending physician. They discovered that he was unhappy with his own diagnosis. Actually, now that he thought about it, the doctor had been surprised that the Creightons died so abruptly. The police then made another discovery: in the short time that her brother had lived with her, Fanny Creighton had persuaded him to invest in a $1,000 life insurance policy, naming her as beneficiary.

Down at the corner store, the owner mentioned that Avery had complained of being constantly fed chocolate pudding at home. No matter how often he told his sister that he was tired of it, she insisted that he eat a little before bed, he had told his boss, slightly baffled by her determination. Both of them had wondered why she was so insistent about the dessert.

Alarmed, the Newark detectives decided to search the house. They didn't find a secret stash of poison. But they did discover that Fanny Creighton's pale clear skin owed something to chemistry. She had a half-empty bottle of Fowler's Solution in the bathroom. It was a popular tonic, available from any druggist. But as any toxicologist knew, it was also an arsenic solution, creating that look of near-translucent skin by a low-level poisoning of the user.

The police promptly hired gravediggers to exhume the boy's body. The belated autopsy and chemical tests found arsenic swirled through every organ. The Newark police arrested Fanny and her husband on suspicion of conspiring to kill the boy, and announced that they planned to dig up both of the elder Creightons as well.

Most chemists considered arsenic detection as the foundation of forensic toxicology. Chemists had learned to find evidence for it in cadavers in the early 1800s, but the results had been troublingly unpredictable. The first truly reliable test dated to 1846, when an outraged English chemist named James Marsh realized that his own flawed test results — based on the somewhat erratic method used at the time — had enabled a poisoner to go free. After being found not guilty, the man had rather mockingly admitted to the crime. Marsh returned to his laboratory and worked like a madman for several years until he had found a way to catch arsenic poisoners.

The Marsh test involved finely mincing suspect tissues, mixing in sulfuric acid, and exposing the bubbling mess to hydrogen gas in a heated tube. If the mixture contained arsenic, the resulting chemical reaction would plaster a gleaming blackish-brown layer on the glass of the tube. Marsh called this an "arsenic mirror," and its dark shine was a sure tell for the metallic poison.

Even in Gettler's day, the Marsh test was still a reliable way to test for arsenic in a corpse. But since Marsh's time chemists had created a catalog of alternative ways to double-check those results. There was the sublimation test, the reduction test, the ammoniosulfate of copper test, the ammonionitrate of silver test, the hydrogen sulfide and hydrochloric acid test, Bettendorf's test, Fleitmann's test, Gosio's test, Berzelius's modification of Marsh's test, and the recently developed Reinsch's test, which scientists hoped would be the most sensitive yet.

In Reinsch's test, the organ under study was decomposed with potassium chlorate (a highly reactive compound of potassium, chlorine, and oxygen) and hydrochloric acid until the tissue dissolved into a yellow liquid. Excess chlorine was boiled away, and the remaining material was first neutralized with ammonia, then made slightly acidic again with more hydrochloric acid. A strip of copper foil was placed into the noxious mixture and left to stand for several hours or even overnight.

The copper strip was then heated. If the tissues had contained a metallic element like arsenic, a dark purplish-gray film would glaze over the hot metal. That was the first part of the process, the first clue. Reinsch's test was tricky because other poisonous elements — antimony, mercury, bismuth, gold, and platinum — could also tarnish the copper strip.

To make sure of the exact poison, a chemist needed to then wash and dry the tarnished strip, put it in a sterile glass tube, and heat the tube over a flame. The heat would cause that thin poisonous film to vaporize and then, as the tube cooled, to deposit a hazy layer on the interior glass.

That final haze provided the real answer. Mercury, for instance, glimmered silvery bright on the glass. Arsenic formed a fine frost, glittering faintly with the octahedral crystals so familiar to chemists who worked with poisons.

John and Fanny Creighton hired one of the best defense attorneys in New Jersey, a former prosecutor named James McCarthy, who wasted no time proclaiming that his clients were innocent; he was "absolutely convinced that they had nothing whatever to do with this thing."

The Creightons had told him they were shocked and baffled to learn that arsenic had been found in the boy's body. Yes, it had been found, but no one knew where it had come from. Charles Avery might even have taken it himself, McCarthy declared. Fanny had told the lawyer that she'd worried about an unhappy love affair. "We are all up in the air," the attorney added. "My clients certainly know nothing about how it came to be there."

Throughout the trial, he hammered that point. The discovery of Fowler's Solution in the household meant nothing; one could find it in thousands of households, used for the most innocent purposes. Fowler's was a very dilute poison anyway — about one part arsenic to one hundred parts liquid. It would take gallons to achieve what Newark chemists said they'd found in the body — arsenic at four times the lethal dose. And there was no evidence, none at all, that either Creighton had suddenly started buying more concentrated arsenic materials.

Rather, the boy himself had easy access to arsenic; he worked in a grocery store, where products like Rough on Rats were stacked high on shelves. Perhaps he was an addict. Dedicated arsenic eaters were known in Europe. In southeastern Austria, peasants reputedly smeared an arsenic paste on toast, folklore asserting that it improved their health and provided a kind of protective poison immunity. "It is not impossible that young Avery carried quantities of arsenic-containing poison around with him," the defense lawyer speculated.

The anonymous letters were evidence of spiteful neighbors, nothing more. The $1,000 insurance policy was a joke; after funeral expenses, there would only be a few hundred left. True, the Creightons routinely outspent their income — John Creighton made only thirty dollars a week as a clerk, after all — but plenty of people were in debt, and they didn't mix poison into the family pudding.

It was ridiculous, McCarthy said, on the face of it.

The prosecutor might have argued that McCarthy was simply offering one alternate theory after another. But even he was forced to acknowledge "the remote possibility that young Avery died of an overdose of arsenic, self-administered."

On June 23 both Creightons — Frances, still in her demure black dress, and her husband — were acquitted of all charges. Journalists who crowded into the Newark courtroom reported that a slight smile appeared on her face and then she fainted into her lawyer's arms. But that wasn't the end of the story, certainly not as far as the prosecutors were concerned. There was still the question of what had happened to John's parents.

Walter and Annie Creighton lay at rest in Newark's Fairmont Cemetery, founded in 1855, 150 stately acres of gentle hills, leafy elm trees, beautifully trimmed firs, and elaborate marble mausoleums. Many of the city's most influential citizens also lay there: Civil War heroes, U.S. congressmen, professional baseball players, Newark mayors, brewery owners, and the founder of the well-established Mennen Company.

The city ordered the couple's bodies exhumed in May, turning the dignified burial grounds into a madhouse of journalistic competition. Police fought a near-military action at the gates, fending climbers with cameras off the walls. One photographer who eluded them and made his way almost to the gravesite was arrested and charged with disorderly conduct.

In desperation, the pathologists decided not even to attempt to move the bodies to the morgue; they erected a rough tent over the gravesite and conducted their autopsies on gurneys. Behind the cloth flaps, using buckets of water to keep their saws and knives clean, they'd cut deep into the decaying bodies. They left unsure exactly what had killed the couple, but they were able to clear up one question: neither Creighton appeared to have died of the diseases listed on the death certificates.

Grimly, the doctors scooped the internal organs into glass jars, placed them into fiber bags, and marched their samples past the shouting reporters. The results were dramatically revealed several weeks later, during the Avery trial: the senior Creighton's body appeared to be clean of poison, but in his wife's body, crystals of white arsenic were discovered.

Just one day after being acquitted of her brother's death, Mary Frances Creighton was rearrested and charged with killing her mother-in-law. The Newark prosecutor did not charge her husband this time — he'd come to suspect that she was the killer in the house. She looked like a lost Madonna, but he could promise any listener that she was nothing of the kind.

That was exactly what prosecutor Victor D'Aloia told the second jury, letting his voice carry through the packed courtroom, through the double wooden doors, into the hall, where the overflow crowd tipped forward, trying to hear. This woman sitting quietly in her black dress and jet-bead necklace was a liar and a murderer, he said.

A nurse who had cared for the elderly Mrs. Creighton testified that the woman had first become ill after her daughter-in-law fixed her a cup of cocoa. The invalid was just recovering when Frances offered to watch over her while the nurse went down to the kitchen for breakfast. When the nurse returned twenty minutes later, the elder Mrs. Creighton's eyes were fixed on the open door, wide and terrified.

"What has happened?" the nurse had cried, hurrying to the bed. Her patient only looked at her, gurgled in her throat, and then vomited onto the floor. The nurse sent an urgent summons to the doctor, and they fought for an hour to save her, but Annie Creighton died late that December morning in 1920.

The physician admitted he hadn't suspected arsenic. Because his patient had been unable to speak, he'd concluded that she'd suffered a cerebral hemorrhage brought on by the violent distress of some kind of food poisoning. Only after the earlier trial, and the carnage in the graveyard, had he realized that her symptoms were consistent with arsenic poisoning.

"I know that Fanny is guiltless of killing my mother," John Creighton told reporters. "If my mother died of unnatural causes I know in my innermost heart that my wife is innocent of responsibility for her death."

Creighton sat behind his wife during the trial, the polished wooden railing between them, listening silently to the sharp discussion of what could be found in a disintegrating body and other debates over chemical detective work.

Prosecutors had called in two prominent

pathologists, Otto Schultz of Columbia University (who had competed for Norris's job in 1918) and Harrison Martland of Newark City Hospital (who had studied at Bellevue), considered one of the best forensic scientists on the East Coast. Both testified that they believed the woman had been killed with white arsenic.

Fanny Creighton's lawyer countered with three New York experts, all from Bellevue and New York University, who methodically tore apart the prosecution case.

The first doctor said he still found the original ptomaine diagnosis most credible; there were too few lesions in the body, he said, to support arsenic poisoning. The second expert, a Bellevue pathologist, said the same thing. He testified that lethal doses would have created the classic internal damage, so visible in the Shelbourne Restaurant deaths, the bloody tracks so characteristic of the poison. In every other case of arsenic poisoning that he'd investigated, "there was always present some or more typical lesions or effects." In this case, he saw none of that predictable damage.

And Gettler, who was the third defense witness, offered a chemist's explanation of why a small amount of arsenic had been found in the body. The New Jersey pathologists had sent samples from the organs to Gettler's lab. They contained a grayish-white powder, Gettler said, which resembled arsenic but was actually the remnant of another element called bismuth. Scattered through the bismuth powder were a few white crystals of arsenic. He was surprised, Gettler told the jury, at how slight was the amount of arsenic found. In the liver, where poisons tended to concentrate, the levels were "infinitesimal."

Gettler had used Reinsch's test, among others, and picked his way through the chemical layers of the analysis to calculate the precise ratios of arsenic and the bismuth in the samples he'd used. As the journalists gloomily reported, these few hours in the courtroom were a long drone of scientific terminology. The chalkboard used to illustrate the conclusions, one reporter said, took on the appearance of an impenetrable spiderweb.

Like arsenic, bismuth was a metallic element used in medicines. In particular, it was a key ingredient in antinausea and antidiarrhea formulas. One of the most popular brands, Bismosal, had been developed in 1901 by a pediatrician seeking to alleviate infant cholera. The solution, wintergreen in taste and colored pink, was renamed Pepto-

Bismol in 1919. Annie Creighton's doctor had not suggested that she take Pepto-Bismol, but he had prescribed another, very similar bismuth formula.

The problem with such formulas, Gettler explained, was that bismuth ore often contained other heavy metals, such as arsenic and lead. Not all processors were able to remove the contaminants; traces of both metals were frequently found in bismuth-based medications. When he ran Reinsch's test, Gettler recognized the characteristic proportions in Annie Creighton's body — large amounts of bismuth and slight traces of arsenic and lead. His conclusion was that the evidence of arsenic poisoning cited by the prosecution was really just evidence of contamination in the medicine prescribed.

For the second time in three weeks, a Newark jury found Fanny Creighton not guilty of murder. She walked out of the courthouse a free woman on July 13, pausing on the steps, smiling at the sound of a hurdy-gurdy playing nearby. She told reporters that she wanted only to be reunited with her children: "I bear no malice toward anyone," she said. "I realize the prosecutor did his duty. I have no plans for the future and I don't know what I shall do. I am too happy with my family just now to think of anything else. But I shall never forget Friday the 13th."

And neither would Alexander Gettler. But it would be twelve years and another arsenic murder trial later before the New York press would start referring to Mary Fanny Creighton as America's Lucretia Borgia. Only then would Gettler — and everyone else — wonder how she'd fooled so many people in the summer of 1923. What Alexander Gettler didn't know then was that July 13, 1923, would haunt him as well.

# FIVE:
# MERCURY (Hg)
## 1923–1925

Charles Webb courted Gertrude Gorman for eight years. He wished to marry her; he had from the beginning. But his chosen sweetheart was the only child of a widowed mother — and her mother couldn't stand him. Gertie's friends dismissed him with contempt: "One of those soft-spoken men you find on the arms of rich women," they said. Her family mocked him; he was dog-like in the way he followed her, an uncle pronounced.

Webb *was* a soft-spoken man, quiet for a New York City estate broker. He was Princeton educated, well read, thoughtful, and as determined as he was gentle-mannered. He shrugged off the hostility and continued his courtship. He was almost fifty — a slight man in shades of gray, with pale eyes and silvering hair — when her mother died in 1920. Gertie was nearly forty then, still the devoted daughter, and the sheltered, bejeweled, fur-draped child of a wealthy and possessive parent. It took Webb two years yet to persuade her to marry him, but they wed at the close of 1922, and he happily moved into her family home on Madison Avenue.

Ten months later his new wife was dead, collapsing in their luxury suite at the Westchester Biltmore Country Club in Rye. And one day after that, on September 28, 1923, her uncle summoned journalists to his country estate in the exclusive enclave of Devon, Pennsylvania. He met them outside, naturally, not wanting newshounds inside his house. Standing in one of the beautifully maintained side gardens, William T. Hunter basked in the floral blaze around him, the dahlias he bred and cultivated as a hobby, the golden petals of a prize-winning bloom that he'd named "Gertie Gorman" for his niece.

The family had been "very much surprised when they heard she intended to marry Webb," he said. They'd thought that she planned to devote her life to her close relatives and friends — she'd always been such a family girl, a "sensible girl." He regretted saying it, but they'd been sadly unsurprised when the marriage killed her. They'd always suspected that Webb had been attracted to more than her sweet ways. What he really loved, her family believed, was the Gorman money. Webb was not a wealthy man, her uncle reminded the gathered journalists; his wife "had all the money." And who wouldn't love a fortune of $2 million (the equivalent of about $25 million today)?

Colonel Hunter didn't directly accuse Webb, not by name anyway, of murder. But there was no missing his intent. "Gertie was given bichloride of mercury to cause her death. That's a bold statement, but there's little doubt in my mind that it's true."

Bichloride of mercury — also known by the unpleasant name of corrosive sublimate — is a poisonous salt of the metallic element mercury. The salt has an uncomplicated chemical structure: one atom of mercury bound tightly to two atoms of chlorine ($HgCl_2$).

In chemistry, though, simplicity doesn't necessarily mean safety. Mercury is a famously risky material. And its neatly arranged salts have proven to be exceptionally poisonous, sometimes even more so than their metallic parent.

Elemental mercury is a slippery substance. In the Earth's crust it anchors itself by bonding with other elements, creating materials such as the rough coppery rock cinnabar, a crystalline combination of mercury and sulfur. Once cinnabar is mined and crushed, mercury can be easily separated from its mineral companions. The warmer aboveground temperatures and the decrease in pressure allow pure mercury to take the form of a very odd liquidlike metal. But unlike a drop of water, a drop of mercury touched by a finger does not wet the skin. Instead, it breaks into smaller drops, tiny glittering balls that skitter away, breaking into ever-smaller balls if touched again. That brilliant scatter effect prompted alchemists to nickname the metal "quicksilver" and to formally name it Mercury, for the fleet-footed Roman messenger god.

The same silver-sphere formation also explains why mercury is less acutely dangerous in its purest form. High surface tension keeps the fluid metal balled up, preventing it from puddling outward, as a traditional liquid would, or from readily soaking into its environment. That same self-containing tension also keeps pure mercury from being easily absorbed by the body.

A few people, mostly in the mid-nineteenth century, had actually swallowed a gleaming cupful, believing it would cure constipation. But the element mostly slipped right through. The mercury drinkers showed no signs of acute sickness, although many complained of developing extremely sore mouths. Neither does elemental mercury absorb easily through skin. Those spherical droplets tend to just jitter over the surface ridges on fingers rather than soak into the tissue. No one has ever called elemental mercury harmless, though. The mercury drinkers of the ninteenth century didn't necessarily become sick immediately, but many later developed cancers, referred to as "mercurial tumors" in the medical textbooks of the time.

Mercury salts work faster and cause more immediate injury, largely because living tissues tend to soak up salty liquids. And mercury bichloride is basically just another chlorine-based salt, a mean-tempered cousin of the familiar sodium chloride (NaCl) that we use as table salt. It's the absorption factor that makes mercury salts so famously dangerous. These quicksilvered compounds dissolve readily in water or alcohol and spread rapidly through living tissues. As medical accounts of the 1920s noted, mercury bichloride was so corrosive, so irritating, that it could destroy tissue to the point that teeth loosened in the mouth, and the stomach eroded into a mass of bleeding ulcers. Physicians knew that because mercury salts, despite the risks, were available in an astonishing variety of commercial products.

Mercury compounds were sold as bedbug killers. They came mixed into laxatives, antiseptics, and diuretics. In extreme cases, doctors prescribed them for chronic bacterial infections such as syphilis. At the time when Gertie Webb's uncle was making his accusations, both the benefits and the murderous potential of mercury bichloride were well known. The poison's risky attributes had been impressed on film fans everywhere, thanks to a Hollywood-fueled tabloid scandal of 1920.

It was the irresistibly tragic tale of a beautiful young actress, the adventure-loving heroine of one successful film after another: *Madcap Madge, The Flapper,* and — what would turn out to be her last picture — *Everybody's Sweetheart.*

The actress, Olive Thomas, had the look of a charming child, with a shining bob of curly dark hair, big violet-blue eyes, and a pale, heart-shaped face. The look launched her career, starting in 1914 when she'd won a "Most Beautiful Girl in New York City" contest. She went on to become a featured Ziegfeld dancer at the New Amsterdam

Theatre, a graceful waif, drifting in a zephyr of scarves. The pin-up artist Alberto Vargas painted her wearing only a red rose and a wisp of black satin. Within a few years she was making films for the Selznick studios.

In the way of people whose lives seem charmed, Thomas soon married a member of the Hollywood's elite, Jack Pickford, younger brother of screen star Mary Pickford. The couple rapidly developed a reputation for wild behavior, intense partying, and intense quarreling, usually over his numerous affairs — he'd developed syphilis as a result of one of them. They separated, reunited, separated, and tried again, delighting the gossip magazines. "She and Jack were madly in love with one another but I always thought of them as a couple of children playing together," Mary Pickford observed sadly in her autobiography many years later.

In early September 1920 the couple sailed to Paris, reportedly on a reconciliation holiday. They checked into the Hotel Ritz and whirled off to enjoy the Prohibition-free city, drinking and dancing at Left Bank bistros until the early morning. At the end of one particularly drunken spree, Pickford and Thomas staggered into their hotel room at nearly three in the morning. Jack, barely standing, fell into the bed. His wife, still energized by the adventure, puttered around the room, wrote a letter, and, finally tiring, went into the bathroom to get ready for sleep.

As Pickford told the police, he was floating in a whiskeyed haze when Olive began screaming, over and over, "Oh my god, my god." He stumbled into the dimly lit bathroom, where she was leaning against the counter. Mistaking it for her sleeping medicine, she had picked up a bottle of the bichloride of mercury potion that he rubbed on his painful syphilis sores, poured a dose, and chugged it down. As the corrosive sublimate burned down her throat, she had a moment to realize her mistake. He caught her up and carried her back to the bed, grabbing the phone and calling for an ambulance. "Oh my god," she repeated, "I'm poisoned."

As the story broke, as Thomas lingered in the hospital for three more days, the newspapers repeated every rumor smoking around them: Pickford's infidelities had driven her to suicide; he had wished to get rid of her and tricked her into taking the poison. As the days passed, he became more evil, she more saintly. So many people flocked to Thomas's funeral in Paris that women fainted in the crush and the streets became carpeted with countless hats, knocked off and trampled.

The police launched an investigation, including an autopsy, and concluded that it was, as Pickford had said, just a terrible accident. In an interview with the *Los Angeles Examiner* after his return to California, Pickford dwelled on how much his wife had wanted to live: "The physicians held out hope for her until the last moment, until they found her kidneys paralyzed. Then they lost hope. But the doctors told me she had fought harder than any patient they ever had."

Olive Thomas's demise, for all the feverish attention it received, was actually a rather standard death from bichloride of mercury. In New York City the medical examiner's office calculated that the compound caused about twenty deaths a year, mostly suicides and similarly unfortunate accidents. But Thomas had definitely given the poison a new star status, at least for the moment.

Gertie Webb's uncle had publicly hinted that the same poison that ended the life of Olive Thomas killed his niece. His accusation seemed, at first, a purely spiteful act, but the authorities were becoming curious.

"There is doubt as to whether or not she died a natural death," the Westchester County coroner admitted to reporters clustered in Rye that September 1923. Her physician had refused to sign a death certificate. In response, the coroner had ordered an autopsy and asked that her viscera be removed and sent to Alexander Gettler in New York City, citing the growing reputation of the toxicology work there.

In late August Charles and Gertie Webb had come to vacation at the Westchester Country Club, bearing a letter of introduction from a club member. The resort catered specifically to their social set. The building was designed in the style of one of Britain's great houses, located on almost six hundred acres of land owned by the Commodore and Biltmore Hotel Company. It offered ponds for fishing, an eighteen-hole golf course, turquoise-tiled pools, tennis courts, card games in the parlors, tea dances, and a private beach club a short distance away.

Gertie's mother had enjoyed the luxury hotel life as well, taking her daughter every summer to old-money resorts in Bridgeport, Connecticut. Webb had persuaded his new wife to try a different place; the old ones, with all their memories, made her melancholy. In August they'd arrived in Rye, planning to do nothing much but play tennis in the day, dance in the evening, and play cards at night. But within a week Gertie was complaining of pain in her side and shortness of breath. Webb summoned a highly recommended doctor staying nearby, William Meyer, who diagnosed a case of mild pneumonia.

Meyer served an exclusive wealthy clientele, maintaining offices in nearby White Plains and in an elegant suite on Manhattan's Park Avenue. He also had a favorite hobby: medical detective work. As an amateur criminologist, he regularly gave lectures in Manhattan high schools on the science of crime, especially on discovering concealed murders. To the trained eye, as he told the district attorney, Gertie Webb's illness seemed peculiar from the outset.

A slight case of pneumonia wasn't so alarming in itself, but his patient seemed oddly sicker than she should have been. Meyer hadn't liked the waxy yellow tone to her skin, the breathy weakness of her voice, and the inexplicable way her health worsened under treatment.

Nothing he did seemed to help. Finally, he decided that her illness just couldn't be caused by a natural disease. And in that case he knew whom to blame. He abruptly barred Webb from the sickroom. She died a few days later, but the doctor gave himself credit anyway: "If I hadn't, she wouldn't have lived as long as she did."

In Gettler's laboratory, mercury bichloride was an unhappily familiar substance.

He'd published his first paper on mercuric chloride poisoning in 1917, before he'd become city toxicologist, while he was holding down only one job, as chemist for Bellevue's pathology department.

It wasn't a particularly difficult poison to detect in a body. But Gettler had been experimenting with it in smaller and smaller amounts, pushing the limits of Reinsch's test, following those careful steps of heating, distilling, and condensing it until the pure poison separated out. He tried to improve the sensitivity until he could detect a mere trace.

The final steps in Reinsch's test involved placing a clean strip of copper in a slurry of suspect tissue and acid, waiting to see if mercury formed a glossy film over the probe. Gettler recognized that the longer he waited, the more mercury might build up on that copper probe. If the slurry was high in mercury, the copper strip glossed over quickly. But if he left the strip to stew overnight before proceeding to the next stage — removing the probe and heating it in a clean glass tube — the test was more sensitive. Even if he couldn't see mercury on the copper, he discovered, this final heating could cause that invisible trace to vaporize and condense inside the tube, coating it with a fine, just detectable quicksilver sheen. In fact, the process was so sensitive that Gettler could detect even the minimal evidence left by one measured spoonful of prescription medicine.

He worked with other procedures as well, seeking confirmation. If a poisoned slurry of tissue was exposed to hydrogen sulfide (the noxious gas that gives rotting eggs their smell), the solution would color and discolor in precise order — yellowish-white, then dark yellow, orange, brown, and black. Mercury would also form a glittering layer over gold foil, if the gold was wrapped around zinc and placed in that poisonous brew for several hours. But Reinsch's test was the one that Gettler came to believe most reliable, especially as he continued to refine it. If the copper wire was left overnight, if he curved the glass tubes so that not a drop could escape, the test proved sensitive enough to produce the shimmer of mercury from as little as 1/500,000 of a grain of mercury salts.

Well before Gertie Webb's organs arrived at Bellevue — stomach, kidneys, liver, intestines, all in clean glass containers — Gettler had been analyzing mercury bichloride. He'd learned from every case, from the accidental overdoses and the deliberate ones: the Italian seamstress who swallowed thirty mercury bichloride tablets, the woman who left a note explaining that she was weary of summer heat, the despairing wife who had quarreled once too often with her husband.

None of them had died quickly: as Olive Thomas's case had emphasized, bichloride of mercury did not offer a fast or easy way out. The seamstress, even after swallowing her bottle of pills, had taken two weeks to die. Most of the suicides reviewed by the medical examiner's office lived five to twelve days. Evidence from autopsies suggested that the poison steadily eroded them internally. The organs looked chewed, spattered with bloody lesions, especially the kidneys, which received an excruciatingly high amount of the mercury salts as they struggled to clear the blood.

And so the kidneys were the first place Gettler looked when checking for chemical evidence of mercury poisoning. And in his preliminary analysis of Gertie Webb's kidneys, he found the faint, glistening signature of mercury in the tissue.

Charles Webb — Carl to his friends — was having a lousy month.

He'd lost his wife less than a year into their long-awaited marriage. He'd been publicly accused of murdering her, first through sly hints by her relatives, then more directly by her friends: "Girlhood Friend Charges Murder," ran the *New York Times* headline on October 2, over a story based on yet another cozy press conference, this one held in the living room of a White Plains vacation cottage. The accuser, a woman who had attended private schools in Manhattan with Gertie Webb, told reporters that Carl Webb was a devious man. "Until a short time ago, poor innocent Gertie did not know that she was taking poison, as I and other dear friends believe."

While she was still single, Gertie Gorman had signed a will dividing her considerable property among family, friends, and servants. She possessed plenty to divide: the house on Madison Avenue, a country home in Fairfield, Connecticut, three apartment buildings in Manhattan, several acres of land near the city's northwest border at

189th Street, stock in the Bankers Trust Company and Brooklyn City Railway Company, partnership in a real estate and development company, three automobiles, a fine collection of jewelry, a ruby and diamond lorgnette for use at the opera, a solid gold mesh evening bag, silver, artwork, clothing, and furs of silver fox and sealskin, as well as several hundred thousand dollars in bank accounts.

But after Gertie Webb became ill in Rye, she had signed a far briefer will, only twenty lines long, that left everything to her husband. This, her angry friends and relatives insisted, had been his design. He had forced this will on a dying woman, which they believed was the sole purpose of the marriage. "There will be trouble by the others when it is filed," Webb reportedly told his lawyer, and he was right.

The day after his wife's old friend gave her incendiary press conference, the day he learned that the Westchester County grand jury had been called into session concerning his wife's death, Carl Webb tried, in his quiet manner, to defend himself. He did not call reporters over to visit him at the country club, where he was sheltering. Instead, through his attorney, he released a written statement that began: "I have been naturally reluctant to discuss in the public press the tragedy which has recently befallen me."

He'd wanted time to grieve in private, Webb said, more time than he'd been allowed. "So much publicity, however, has been given to the matter and so many insinuations have been made by persons apparently hostile that my friends have urged me to make a public statement."

Regarding the will — yes, he had filed it for probate. But he also filed a more complex version, unsigned, as a proposed amendment. Gertie had insisted on drafting the short will after she realized how sick she was, he insisted; she'd wanted him to be her beneficiary. He had thought at the time that it gave him too much, so he had asked their attorney to draw up another document that included many of the earlier bequests. But he was unable to get his wife to sign the revised version; for one thing, the doctor had ordered him out of the sickroom.

He hoped to honor its provisions anyway, he said: "My one desire in the matter is to carry out my wife's wishes to the best of my knowledge and ability." As to the accusations, he had no intention of carrying on quarrels in the newspapers. But Webb would say this: he knew nothing about any poison administered to his wife.

Gertie had been completely in the care of Dr. William Meyer during the last three weeks of her life; for part of that time, he — Webb — had been kept entirely out of the sickroom, forced to pray for her recovery in an adjacent sitting room. He'd begged Meyer to bring in other doctors, but the White Plains physician had refused. Webb had himself sent for the doctor she'd once seen at the local hospital, but Meyer had refused to "consult with him or to admit him into the sick room." Webb had then sent his attorney to threaten legal action; Meyer had at last agreed to confer with the Webbs' doctor in New York City and to allow her husband back into the room.

According to Webb's statement, he then waited by her bedside, on his knees, praying, hoping for the other doctor to hurry. But by the time the Manhattan physician arrived, Gertie was dead.

The Westchester district attorney's office, mistrustful of the dramatic performances now being staged in Rye, had not only asked Gettler to handle the toxicology but asked pathologists from the New York City medical examiner's office to do the autopsy.

Once a body is opened up, the presence of mercury bichloride is hard to miss. The kidneys are dribbled with blood, mushy with cellular breakdown, and grayish in color. But there are plenty of other indicators as well: eroded patches in the mouth and throat, ulcerations in the stomach wall, and bloody inflammation of the intestines.

Mercury, for all its glimmering silver elegance, is a messy killer.

The problem — at least for those accusing Charles Webb of murder — was that the Manhattan pathologists didn't find any of that damage in Gertie Webb's body. "All the usual tissue changes in cases of bichloride poisoning were absent," the medical examiner's report concluded. They found no ulceration of the stomach or intestines, no ugly inflammations of the mouth and throat. The doctors did find the lungs congested by pneumonia and the kidneys severely diseased.

For his part, Gettler had been able to estimate the amount of bichloride of mercury in Gertie Webb's body by comparing the Reinsch's test readings with other data that he'd compiled. Mercury was there, but in such minuscule amounts that it was barely detectable, far below a lethal dose. He'd further analyzed the trace of mercury detected, concluding that it wasn't corrosive sublimate at all but rather another mercury compound, one also commonly used but far less toxic.

Gettler identified the mercury source as an old-time remedy called calomel, which was still sometimes used as a laxative or purgative. A familiar tonic, calomel had been prescribed for treating intestinal parasites in the sixteenth century. Lewis and Clark had taken it with them on their explorations of the American West. Doctors still routinely ordered it for patients with gastrointestinal illnesses, using it to flush out the system. It was gradually disappearing though, as physicians realized that it brought the unavoidable risks associated with mercury exposure.

Calomel was, in fact, a milder salt of mercury called mercurous chloride. Its formula was a little different from corrosive sublimate: two mercury atoms for every two chlorine atoms ($Hg_2Cl_2$). The fact that the corrosive chlorine was more tied up meant the preparation was less abrasive; the fact that calomel solutions tended to be much more diluted meant that they were less acutely poisonous.

But like all mercury compounds, they lingered in the body and could accumulate in the tissues. And they naturally concentrated in the kidneys, following the same distribution patterns that characterized the more dangerous bichloride of mercury. To test his theory further, Gettler dosed several cats with calomel at a level comparable to a standard prescription of the medicine. The slight sheen of mercury in their kidneys, he found, was at a similar concentration to what he'd seen in Gertie Webb's organs.

Acting on Gettler's findings, the district attorney began a new round of questioning, reinterviewing Gertie Webb's physicians.

Dr. Meyer hadn't prescribed calomel. Neither had the physicians she'd seen during her hospital visits. But she had been taking regular doses, investigators learned, on the advice of her doctor in Manhattan.

"The only poison in this case, I am convinced, is the slanderous tongues and the evil desires of those who want to make scandal," Webb's attorney snapped to police investigators.

At this point they agreed with him. After the autopsy findings suggested poorly treated diseases might have caused her death, the district attorney had begun investigating Dr. Meyer: "Dr. Meyer was mistaken in thinking he had cured her pneumonic condition. When she died, Mrs. Webb had been suffering from kidney trouble, a bad heart and pleural pneumonia." Her kidney disease, it seemed, had been worsening for some time.

The prosecutor continued the grand jury hearings but required Meyer to waive immunity before testifying, which left him open to criminal charges. Meyer left no doubt as to his feelings: "I took deep personal umbrage . . . the inference given to the grand jury was that I, as attending physician, was not beyond suspicion." He resented even more the implication that he had badgered a dying woman while playing amateur detective.

He admitted that he'd told her that she was dying and that something was killing her but he didn't know what it was. He had asked her if someone could have slipped poison into her coffee or cocoa. She had said no, but he hadn't really believed her. "Remember, Gertie, you are dying," Meyer testified that he'd answered. "It is very important that you tell me everything." When she still had no suspicions, he'd realized that he would have to act for her. He'd felt it was his duty to urge a police investigation. Naturally, he'd shared his information with interested parties such as the dying woman's relatives.

The doctor did not like the way this case was turning out. As Meyer told journalists after the hearing, he didn't care for the district attorney either.

On October 21, the Westchester grand jury announced its findings: Gertie Webb had died of natural causes. The charges against her husband were groundless. "Accusations have been made before this body and through the public press," it said, "which, if true, would seriously affect the status of Charles Webb, husband of the deceased. We, therefore, deem it our duty to say emphatically that all of these accusations are without the slightest foundation and we fully and completely exonerate Mr. Webb." The county coroner backed those findings, issuing a report concluding that Gertie Webb had died of progressive kidney disease and a complicating pneumonia, misdiagnosed by the attending physician.

Webb profusely thanked the district attorney and grand jury for their "strict sense of justice" but also expressed bitterness, stating that he hoped with time the motives of those who had accused him would be fully revealed. He certainly expected to get another chance to find them out. Gertie

Webb's relatives — her father, her uncle, her half brother, and her cousins — had tried to get the governor to overrule the Westchester district attorney. When that had failed, they'd filed a civil suit seeking to overturn her last will.

Being a very public criminal suspect had changed Webb's mind, though, about how to proceed with his wife's last wishes. He decided to withdraw the amended will he'd drafted, the one sharing her property with friends and relatives.

For obvious reasons, as his lawyer said, Carl Webb had lost the impulse to share.

The Webb case showcased a point that Norris had tried to impress on the city police department. He wanted the officers, from detectives to beat cops, to value scientific evidence, to think of the medical examiner's office as a useful partner in an investigation. Earlier that year he'd given a keynote address, "The Medical Examiner and the Police," during the opening ceremonies of the School for Detectives of the City of New York, the first time a scientist had participated in that program.

In the fall of 1923 he'd begun regular training programs for city detectives. He brought them to the morgue, had them attend autopsies, and sent them to Gettler's laboratory. There they could watch the city toxicologist — and the New York University students he was training — work their way through poison analyses of bodies brought in from the street.

Detection of poisons such as mercury bichloride, arsenic, and cyanide formed the routine of Gettler's laboratory. For all the mystery novelists' fascination with more exotic toxins — the British writer Agatha Christie, for instance, launched her career in 1920 with a tale of strychnine and murder — the everyday poisons kept the city toxicology laboratory occupied.

But in the chilly January of 1924 Gettler and his crew got a true oddball case: the death of the famous Blue Man. The victim had spent most of his adult life as a human curiosity exhibited at Barnum and Bailey's (the Greatest Show on Earth) as it traveled around the country. The Blue Man had recently died at Bellevue; the pathologists said his body was one of the strangest they'd ever seen stretched out on a marble table in the morgue.

The famed human oddity was sixty-eight years old when he checked himself into the hospital, short of breath and complaining that when he lay flat he couldn't breathe at all. As his hospital records noted, he was a tall, thin man, with glistening white hair and an equally glossy white mustache. His skin was so deeply blue as to appear black at a distance. His lips were blue; his tongue was blue. The scleras — what would usually be called the whites of his eyes — were also blue.

His wasn't the exhausted bluish patchiness of cyanide poisoning, though. The skin was smoothly colored, with an almost lustrous look. It was that overall effect of polishing that led the doctors to a diagnosis — the Blue Man was suffering from a disease called argyria (from the Greek word *argyros* meaning silver). The condition was known to deposit silver through the body, staining the tissues to a deeply polished blue-gray.

The Bellevue doctors suspected that the Blue Man, a former British army officer, had achieved fame by dosing himself with silver nitrate. This salt, made by dissolving silver into nitric acid and evaporating the solution, formed a shiny powder that could be mixed for other uses. Silver nitrate was easily available: used in photographic processing, in dentistry to treat ulcers in the mouth, and in neonatal care, blended into drops that went into the eyes of newborns to prevent infections.

The Blue Man had firmly denied any silver exposure, denied any self-medication at all. As he'd told his circus admirers, he was a freak of nature, blue at birth. But when he died that fall — from rapidly worsening pneumonia — the pathologists had decided to take a thorough look. The autopsy showed that he was blue-silver on the inside too. The dull reddish-brown muscle tissue had a faint silver tint, the spleen was colored a bluish red, the liver bluish gray. Even the brain shone silver, its familiar curves and coils slightly reflective in the brightly lit morgue.

How much metal did his body contain? To find out, Gettler made an acid solution of the organs and cooked it dry, creating a gray ash. He flushed hot water, ammonia, and nitric acid through the ashes, washing the silver out of them. He then measured the silver from each organ and totaled up the results to calculate the whole body content. Gettler's conservative estimate was that the Blue Man's body contained a good three and a half ounces of solid silver. About half the metal was in the muscle tissue, another fourth in the bones, and the rest mostly concentrated in the liver, kidneys, heart, and brain.

But the silver hadn't killed the Blue Man; he had died of the pneumonia. The only effect the silver doses seemed to have had was to turn him that remarkable indigo color. "Among the heavy metals which may become deposited in the human body in relatively large amounts," Gettler wrote in his report on the case, "silver is of slight and perhaps least toxicity."

Of course, the toxicology lab was now in possession of a nice quantity of pure silver. His co-workers took the gleaming pellets acquired from the Blue Man's body, melted them down, shaped them into a bullet, and gave it to Gettler. Just in case, his friends assured him, he ever had to analyze a vampire.

He put it on his desk. Just in case, he replied.

Charles Webb was still fighting with his dead wife's family a year after being cleared of murder charges. He'd won the first round in this new fight; a judge had ruled that the twenty-line will was valid. Her relatives had appealed that finding, and in July 1924 they filed another lawsuit, insisting that the family home on Madison Avenue was meant to stay in the Gorman family. They also wanted a $250,000 trust fund to maintain the property.

Webb didn't want the house, didn't even live there anymore. He'd moved into a residential hotel. But he'd learned that he wasn't a forgiving man. He went back to court to challenge that claim as well. If it took years, he would make sure that he gave her family nothing, nothing at all.

A case like that of Charles Webb, when science could exonerate an innocent man, was more than gratifying. It emphasized, as Norris had told the police, that forensic research was gaining its place as an investigator's tool. It showcased the way a medical examiner's work could be used to protect people from harm.

But some poisons still challenged their very young science, warning the researchers against overconfidence. In 1924 the New York City medical examiner's office encountered just such a poison, and the experience did not prove so gratifying as that of the Webb case. This new poison emphasized instead the limits of the science, the obstacles that even good chemists and crusading public officials faced, in protecting the public against the new generation of chemicals, desired by industry and promoted by a cooperative government.

The story of this poison did not begin in New York City — although Norris and Gettler would soon enough become involved in investigating its dangers. It began in the Standard Oil Refinery in Elizabeth, New Jersey.

The factory looked harmless enough from the outside, a typical brick building with narrow windows set in stone. Inside, the familiar sounds of work — the hiss and clank of the pipes, the grumble and clatter of the retorts — could be heard. But then came the unfamiliar — a smell carried by vapors rising from the machinery, not the usual odor of gasoline but the dull, musty scent of tetraethyl lead.

Five years earlier a chemical engineer working for General Motors had discovered that tetraethyl lead cured a stubborn knocking problem in car engines. Even GM's best cars, including its elegant Cadillacs, had banged so loudly under the hood that it sounded to customers as if the engines were breaking apart. The noise was a by-product of the engine's design, which involved a somewhat inefficient combustion process. This meant that the gasoline fuel was never completely burned away; the remnants of gasoline tended to heat, ignite, and explode, sometimes loudly enough to startle a driver into losing control.

Tetraethyl lead — or TEL, in industrial shorthand — solved that problem. The compound was actually a nineteenth-century discovery from European laboratories. But a GM engineer, one Thomas Midgley Jr., saw a new use for it, building on research done by a scientific colleague, Charles Kettering. Both men realized that tetraethyl lead (a chemical blending of lead, carbon, and hydrogen) essentially smoothed out the rough patches in gasoline combustion. As the engine churned and burned fuel, the circulating lead formula and its by-products bonded with gasoline remnants that hadn't ignited, buffering them over into nonexplosive materials. The innovative Midgley — he would later develop the chloro-fluorocarbon coolant called Freon — tinkered with the formula until he felt he had just the right TEL mixture for gasoline going into motor vehicles.

The additive was made in the "looney gas building," the employee nickname for Standard Oil's TEL processing plant. In the twelve months since the company began making the antiknock ingredient, plant laborers' fear of the place had steadily increased. The men who worked there, in the clanking heat and drifting vapors, had become a little odd — moody, short-tempered, unable to sleep. They'd started getting lost on the familiar plant grounds, sometimes had trouble remembering their friends. And then in September 1924 the workers started collapsing, going into convulsions, babbling deliriously. By the end of October, thirty-two of the forty-nine TEL workers were in the hospital, and five had died.

Standard Oil issued a cool response: "These men probably went insane because they worked too hard," according to the building manager. And those who didn't survive had merely worked themselves to death. Other than that, the company didn't see a problem.

The statement failed to impress the State of New Jersey, which ordered the plant closed. The local district attorney wasn't impressed either. He called Charles Norris and asked to borrow his toxicologist for some independent research into the chemistry brewed in the hated building.

Norris was pleased to accommodate that request. He hadn't liked Standard Oil's statement and had decided, in fact, to issue his own, explicitly contradicting the industry's perspective on TEL: "The fact that it is readily absorbed and highly poisonous was discovered in Germany about 1854 when tetraethyl lead was discovered, and it has not been used in industry during most of its seventy years since then because of its known deadliness."

Investigators discovered that before the illnesses at Standard Oil, another TEL processor, the Dupont Company, had lost two workers at its Dayton, Ohio, plant. They had died from lead poisoning. Lead is well known for its tendency to damage the nervous system. And lead-laced vapors, like those emitted in TEL manufacturing, are absorbed through the skin and inhaled directly into the lungs. Months before the New Jersey workers died, several of the supervisors at the "looney gas building" had actually recommended that production be shut down.

In answer to this new round of criticisms, Standard Oil went straight to the source. It brought in Midgley, the TEL developer, to hold a press conference at its Manhattan offices. He assured reporters that handled properly there was nothing dangerous about his prize discovery. To prove it, he washed his hands in a bowl filled with TEL. "I'm taking no chances whatever," he said. "Nor would I take any chances by doing that every day."

The management at Dupont and Standard Oil blamed the workers for failing to protect themselves. Gloves and masks had been available at the refinery. It was the workers' responsibility to wear them. But they weren't well-educated men, a company vice president explained to the reporters, and may not have realized that working with TEL was "man's work," with all the risks implied.

It took Gettler a full three weeks to figure out how much tetraethyl lead the Standard Oil workers had absorbed before they became ill, crazy, or dead. The compound was so rarely used, so new in American industrial production, that there were no readily available tests or much background information.

Two years earlier the U.S. Public Health Service had asked Midgley for a record of all research into the health consequences of TEL. He'd replied that no such research existed, and since then neither Dupont, GM, Standard Oil, nor the federal government had spent much time evaluating the compound.

"This is one of the most difficult of many difficult investigations of the kind which have been carried on at this laboratory," Norris said. "This was the first work of its kind, as far as I know. Dr. Gettler had not only to do the work but to invent a considerable part of the method of doing it."

Working with the first four bodies, then checking his results against the body of the last worker killed, who had died screaming in a straitjacket, Gettler discovered that the TEL and its lead by-products form a recognizable distribution pattern, concentrating in the lungs, the brain, and the bones. The highest amounts were spread through the lungs, indicating that most of the poison had been somehow inhaled; later tests showed that the masks used by Dupont and Standard Oil did not filter out the lead in TEL vapors.

Rubber gloves did protect the hands, but if TEL splattered and made any direct contact with the skin, it was absorbed extremely quickly. A few months after his press conference, Thomas Midgley Jr. left for an extended European vacation, seeking treatment for the effects of lead poisoning. As the press speculated, the inventor was either a liar or a daredevil — or perhaps he'd just inhaled too much "looney gas."

After Norris released his office's report on tetraethyl lead, New York City banned its sale and the sale of "any preparation containing lead or other deleterious substances" as an additive to gasoline. So did New Jersey. So did the city of Philadelphia. Afraid that the trend would accelerate, that they would be forced to find another antiknock compound, and that they would lose money on their investment, the manufacturing companies demanded that the federal government take over the investigation and develop its own regulations.

Dupont and Standard Oil agreed to suspend TEL production and distribution until a federal investigation was completed. In May 1925 the U.S. Surgeon General called a national tetraethyl lead conference, to be followed by the formation of a task force to conduct the investigation. The government promised that the scientists assembled would be efficient and finish the study by year's end. The pro-business administration, under Republican President Calvin Coolidge, also made its own position obvious, at least to anyone who'd been following the story.

Norris had persuaded the New York City health commissioner to issue that initial ban on TEL-laced gasoline, writing with his usual directness: "its use should be prohibited, for lead is going to be deposited in the machines and in closed spaces especially. It may be extremely dangerous to have gasoline containing this substance even in small amount."

The government-approved TEL task force did not include Charles Norris or Alexander Gettler — nor anyone from any city where sales of the gas had been banned, or any agency involved in that first critical analysis of tetraethyl lead.

Gettler went back to his usual routine, once again investigating a bichloride of mercury case. That same May, a twenty-one-year-old White Plains woman had been rushed to the hospital after eating a fig from a box that her grandmother had sent her as a gift. The sick girl had been carried into treatment still clutching the box of fruit.

Doctors recognized signs of an acute poisoning — the skin of her mouth was corroded, and she was vomiting blood. The hospital sent the figs directly to the medical examiner's office. The next day Gettler reported that he'd found a silvery-white powder rubbed into the fruit. The figs were loaded with mercury bichloride.

Detectives discovered that the grandmother had quarreled with the young woman's parents over money. The daughter had supported her parents and refused to visit her grandmother again; her six-year-old brother had continued to visit. The older woman evidently regarded her granddaughter's behavior as a deep betrayal. She had bought the figs, laced a basketful with mercury bichloride, and given it to the boy, telling him it was a gift for his sister and "not to eat any himself."

When detectives came to arrest the grandmother, she'd been waiting for them. "All right" was all she said, as she gathered up her handbag and hat. She was lucky, they told her — the girl would recover, and the charge would be only attempted murder. She didn't answer them.

By the end of summer, Norris found himself suffering from a rare exhaustion, worn down by the press of bodies piling up in his department.

July had seen another death caused by hydrogen cyanide gas. It had been used to fumigate a leather storage facility. The gas then seeped through cracks in the wall and killed a man working in his shop next door. Gettler and Assistant Medical Examiner Thomas Gonzales visited with business owners, trying to persuade them to use a different fumigant. Norris also went to the health commissioner and asked him to ban the use of cyanide gas for extermination purposes in New York City.

Its use should be eliminated in every state, Norris said. He strongly suspected the risks were greatly underestimated, that many "heart disease" cases in smaller cities were actually fumigation deaths. But those cities had no trained pathologists at hand to argue the case. New York did, and officials should take advantage of that, he said. This time the health commissioner agreed. After reviewing the records, he issued an official ban on the use of cyanide fumigation in the city.

Norris might be stymied in persuading the federal government to better regulate poisons, but he could at least make a difference in his own city. He had learned to celebrate small victories too.

Still, the number of poison alcohol deaths continued to rise. The Bellevue morgue was seeing an average of two alcohol-poisoned bodies a day. Liquor syndicates were importing pure wood alcohol from Germany, leading Norris to issue yet another warning: "I hope it is understood that the purer the wood alcohol is, the deadlier it is."

Bootlegger street shootings continued unabated. So did fatal illuminating gas accidents, and lethal automobile crashes in the city streets. And "we have been swamped with unknown floaters and unknown babies," Norris wrote to the health department, explaining why he had been slow in issuing death certificates. "It has been almost impossible for us to keep up with our work. Sometimes we have had as many as 15 to 18 cases in a morning at the Morgue, with 9 or 10 autopsies."

In July he decided to take his first vacation in seven years. Or kind of a vacation. He was going to a spa in Europe for treatment of exhaustion.

At the end of 1925, Charles Webb was again in court to fend off his dead wife's relatives' demands for money. And he would be there again. And again. Not for another three years would all the legal actions be settled, giving him clear title to Gertie's estate. She'd not been as rich as the rumors had it. Rich enough, though — the courts set the total value of her estate at $1,033,765,

about half of what speculation had indicated.

Webb received about $630,000 of it: most
on the remainder went to paying his legal
fees and court costs. He never moved back
into the home he'd shared with Gertie; he
sold the house and spent the rest of his
years in a New York apartment. He continued to run a real estate company. But once
the court battles were over, and the inheritance came to him, he set about keeping a
promise he had made to his dying wife.
She'd wanted a park in New York City as a
memorial to her mother.

Webb donated the empty plot she'd owned
on the city's Upper West Side. It comprised
almost two acres of rolling land in Washington Heights — a nice little stretch between
West 189th and West 190th streets, along
the edge of Broadway as it ran north
through the city. In addition to the land —
which the city valued at $300,000 — Webb
gave another $25,000 for a playground and
$50,000 for a maintenance fund.

The new park was designed in a series of
terraces, descending toward Broadway. A
central stairway, constructed of stone, led to
walking paths, which in turn meandered
through shady sitting areas. Along one edge,
Webb ordered the construction of a silvery

stone wall. Embedded in the stone, he had placed a small plaque dedicating the park to Gertie A. Gorman. It was — and is — a beautiful little park. But it also stands for an end, a closure, and, most of all, a tribute to someone loved and lost.

# Six:
# Carbon Monoxide
# (CO), Part I

## 1926

In late January 1926, a snow-sprayed wind glittering around him, a reporter from the *New York Times* shivered on a certain street corner, the one an irate letter writer had described as the noisiest in Manhattan — "the nadir of quietness." At the designated intersection, Sixth Avenue and 34th Street, the journalist attempted to interview a traffic cop about that complaint. But the reporter worried that his task might be impossible. As he later wrote, while he could see the officer's lips moving, he couldn't hear a word of the answer.

"Bang, flop, bang, flop. A flat-wheeled surface car jolted its way over the tracks, with every nut and every bolt protesting. Blah! Blah! Blah!!! Went the semi-siren of a lumbering truck," he wrote, trying to re-create the blast of sound around him. The vehicular rush ran so thickly here, the city had assigned six officers to the one corner.

The reporter had simply picked the police-man he could see best, the tallest of traffic guardians. The two men surveyed the chaos of automobiles before them: Maxwell Traveling Sedans, Dodge Brothers limousines, Packard's new six-cylinder touring sedans, Nash Specials, Chandler Metropolitans, the occasional Jordan Victoria, Willys Knight's compact four-passenger coupe, stretched-out Cadillac Suburbans, sporty Buick Country Club Specials, and Ford Model Ts, a motorized stampede of mostly black, boxy vehicles, some in the old open design, many with the new flat roofs, all with blaring horns and round staring-eye headlamps.

"Hey," the police officer shouted at a speeding driver. "He put his whistle between his lips and presumably blew it," the reporter noted. Nine more motorized vehicles went by, sixty-nine pedestrians, two baby carriages, and three more surface cars — the name for streetcars, to distinguish them from the railcars screeching overhead on the elevated tracks.

The traffic cop leaned down and put his lips to the writer's left ear: "It's the noisiest place in the world."

Other policemen might have argued for that honor, at other street corners, in countless other cities. Traffic jammed intersections across the country, bred by the automobile craze of the 1920s. Everyone wanted a car — for the speed, the independence, and yes, the status. Four million new cars had been sold nationwide in 1925, and automobile manufacturers predicted with absolute confidence that those numbers could only rise. The National Automobile Show, held at Manhattan's Grand Central Palace, showcased more than five hundred new models in 1926 — bigger cars, more powerful cars, cars riding on the new, cushier balloon tires. Cheaper cars. The Dodge brothers (Horace and John) had reduced the price of their luxury Type A sedan from $1,280 to $1,045, in an effort to lure more customers.

In New York City a personal automobile offered escape from standing on a snowslushed sidewalk waiting for a surface car, and from risking one's life in the rackety elevated trains. Reliable public transportation had yet to be realized; Mayor Hylan blamed strong resistance and political lobbying by private transportation companies: "Let the people know that selfishness is still rampant in this city." At party headquarters these denunciations of lucrative donors were not appreciated. In 1926 he was replaced as mayor by Tammany Hall's new favorite, the luxury- and limousine-loving James J. Walker.

Even Charles Norris had developed car fever.

His examiners had been taking taxis to death scenes. They'd wasted hours waiting for those city-chartered cabs, and more hours walking, after the cars failed to start. "I understand that the taxicabs at present time are in very poor condition" and are constantly breaking down, Norris wrote to the city's transportation manager. Please, could some cars be permanently assigned to the medical examiner's office? He could make do with a meager two.

Norris received an apologetic refusal; the city had no cars to spare at the moment. The new mayor's office was using them all.

Frustrated, Norris turned his own private car, and chauffeur, over to department use. He did persuade Bellevue to pay the chauffeur's $1,000-a-year salary. The driver was as necessary as the car itself, as most of Norris's city-born employees didn't know how to drive. For that matter, it seemed, neither did the people who were, at the moment, careening around Sixth Avenue in their newly purchased automobiles.

In 1920 the medical examiner's office tallied 692 people killed by automobiles in New York City; five years later that number was 1,272, despite a state law, passed in 1922, that required drivers to be licensed. Both Norris and the Manhattan district attorney, Joshua Banton, had worked hard to get the licensing law passed. Their joint public position was brief and completely clear: "There are many persons driving automobiles in this city who ought not to drive."

The motorized stampede pressured the federal government to resolve the risk posed by lead additives to gasoline. In January 1926 the Public Health Service released its report on tetraethyl lead, concluding that there was "no danger" in adding the compound to gasoline, and no reason to prohibit the sale of leaded gasoline as long as workers were well protected during the manufacturing process.

The scientists who wrote the report had been recruited by both the government and industry. They'd studied the risks associated with everyday exposure by drivers, automobile attendants, and gas station operators and found it to be minimal. True, all the drivers tested showed trace amounts of lead in their blood. But a low level of lead could be tolerated, the scientists believed; none of the test subjects showed the extreme behaviors and breakdowns associated with the "looney gas building."

Critics, even then, charged that the panel was biased, deliberately underestimating the risks. But, in fact, the conclusions weren't entirely wrong: the extra protections recommended for industrial workers did make the factories safer. Workers exposed to TEL at lower levels did not drop to the ground or show immediate signs of ill health. Workers who were well buffered against the additive were not rushed to the hospital or strapped into straitjackets. There was no arguing with the report's finding that safety precautions did the job.

The federal panel did issue one cautionary note however: exposure levels would probably rise as more and more people took to the road. Perhaps at a later point, the scientists suggested, the research should be taken up again. It was always possible that leaded gasoline might "constitute a menace to the general public after prolonged use or other conditions not foreseen at this time."

But that was the future's problem. In 1926, citing evidence from the TEL report, the federal government revoked all bans on the production and sale of leaded gasoline.

The reaction of industry was jubilant; one Standard Oil spokesman likened the compound to a "gift of God," so great was its potential to improve automobile performance.

Toxicologists like Alexander Gettler had more urgent worries about risks in the age of the automobile: focusing on other chemicals released in engine exhaust. When gasoline or any other carbon-rich fuel burned in the modern engine, a cascade of reactions resulted, atoms separating and recombining, loose carbon bonding with circulating oxygen. Those carbon-and-oxygen connections, in particular, created two differently troublesome gases: carbon dioxide and carbon monoxide.

In general, when fuel combustion is highly efficient, the main by-product is carbon dioxide — a single carbon atom attached to two oxygen atoms. No scientist really considers carbon dioxide a poison, not in the routine sense of the word. It is a natural by-product of the human metabolic process, among other things. When people breathe, inhale air, they take in oxygen, then exhale back out carbon dioxide (created in the carbon-rich interior of humans and other animals).

Carbon dioxide ($CO_2$) occasionally killed directly in the 1920s, but rarely. Such deaths occurred when $CO_2$ displaced oxygen in a tightly closed space. In transporting fruits and vegetables, for example, shippers often kept the produce cold with superchilled carbon dioxide. At about 103 degrees below zero Fahrenheit, the gas freezes to a solid, turning into glassy-looking chunks of exceptionally cold material. As the chunks warm and "melt," they return directly to a gaseous state, giving the material the nickname "dry ice." In an unventilated space, this seeping release of carbon dioxide will gradually replace oxygen, suffocating anyone inside.

Five longshoremen were once found dead in the cargo hold of a steamer docked in Brooklyn on the East River. The boat had been carrying cherries from Michigan, preserved in a chamber kept chilled with dry ice; the boat workers had been bunking in the room where the fruit was stored. Norris's office found that the men's blood was "saturated with carbon dioxide and the men had obviously died from asphyxia." Hastily taken air samples had confirmed that the room was saturated with the gas.

But as the pathologists emphasized, they'd had to move quickly before the gas was diluted. Carbon dioxide is always found in human blood; and it rises to unusually high levels with other forms of suffocation as well. So carbon-dioxide-rich air samples were essential to determining the method of suffocation. "Exactly the same autopsy picture would have been found if the men had died from being smothered by holding, say, a pillow over their mouths," one of the medical examiners noted later in his memoir.

"This brings up a rather interesting possibility for a method of murder that would be extremely difficult to detect," the doctor, Edward Marten, continued. "I pass this on, for what it is worth, to writers of detective stories." In his scenario, a sleeping or heavily intoxicated person slumbers in bed. The killer places a bucket, packed with dry ice, on the floor and carefully shuts the windows and door as he leaves. Within a few hours the victim suffocates. When someone opens the door, normal air refills the room, whisking away all trace of the murder weapon: "The trick is that when dry ice evaporates it leaves absolutely no trace behind, so that the investigating detectives would find nothing except a dry and completely empty pail." Still, Marten considered that a better tip for fiction writers than for real-life killers. The purchase of dry ice was easy to track, the material was tricky to handle, and the gas was rarely and unreliably deadly.

On the other hand, carbon monoxide proved an exceptionally reliable killer.

Carbon monoxide (CO) is also largely an industrial by-product. When fuel does not burn cleanly away, the process is called incomplete combustion. This less efficient use of fuel makes less oxygen available, creating a situation where, frequently, each atom of carbon bonds with only one atom of oxygen, a connection multiplied millions of times over.

CO is relatively rare in nature — it forms in the wake of lightning strikes, forest and grass fires, and any event that causes a carbon-rich fuel to burn. Once in the atmosphere, it tends to attach to other free oxygen, converting to carbon dioxide and dispersing. Still, as a 1923 toxicology text noted, it is always present "to a more or less extent wherever man lives and works."

The gas was first synthesized by a French chemist, who in 1776 heated zinc oxide with coke (a concentrated form of coal). He'd watched the coke ignite with a beautiful blue-violet flame, a color that scientists would later realize was a signature of carbon monoxide as it burned.

Carbon monoxide drifted out of lime kilns, brick kilns, charcoal kilns, burning buildings, stoves, grates, braziers, salamanders (broilers), coal-stoked furnaces, gas-water heaters, gas lighting, the smokestacks of trains, and of course, the tailpipes of automobiles. Auto exhaust contained up to 25 percent carbon monoxide, according to tests done in 1926. An even more concentrated source, though, was illuminating gas. This fuel, produced from coal processing, consisted mostly of carbon monoxide and hydrogen. Illuminating gas was preferred for lighting because it produced a particularly bright flame, but it was also used to power stoves, heaters, and even refrigerators. Some of these appliances had registered gas leaks containing more than 40 percent carbon monoxide.

The risks associated with inhaling high levels of carbon monoxide had been realized quickly, mostly because they made themselves so apparent. Consider the effect of even a small car, a 22-horsepower Model T, left running in a closed garage. An engine that size generated twenty-eight liters of carbon monoxide a minute. Some toxicologists calculated that "this is sufficient to render the atmosphere of a single car garage deadly within five minutes, if the engine is run with the door closed." The federal government issued a more conservative estimate of ten minutes.

Charles Norris estimated that carbon monoxide killed nearly a thousand residents of New York City every year. Breaking Norris's numbers down further — say, for the single year 1925 — his records showed 618 accidental carbon monoxide deaths, 388 suicides, and three homicides. The most inventive of the murders involved a man killed by having a gas tube forced into his mouth until the carbon monoxide killed him. The killer then put the dead man into a water-filled bathtub and reported his death as an accidental drowning.

Unfortunately for the murderer, the man's lungs contained no water. And when Gettler ran the toxicology tests, evidence of carbon monoxide almost literally spilled out of the blood.

Most carbon monoxide murders involved faking an accident. The standard approach was to blame the death on a leaky heater or poorly closed gas valve, setting it up as just another of the many sad fatalities in the city. Both police and medical examiners acknowledged that these crimes were often difficult to detect, and undoubtedly some murderers were never caught.

But law enforcement officials had exposed enough of these schemes to warn against homicidal overconfidence.

One such success, which would be cited by forensic scientists for years following, occurred in the fall of 1923. An out-of-work painter named Harry Freindlich took out a $1,000 life insurance policy on his twenty-eight-year-old wife Leah, smothered her while she lay sleeping, and then attempted to cover it up.

Freindlich was desperate for money at the time, desperate about everything: he was jobless and unable to pay the rent, much less provide food for his family. The family home was a bare cut above living on the street anyway, a battered tenement on Manhattan's Lower East Side. The paint was peeling off the walls. The floors were splintered. They'd been patching the appliances together with cardboard, glue, solder, anything. It was one of these cracked appliances that gave him the idea — a gaslight in the bedroom with a troublesome broken fitting that he had soldered back together more than once.

On an early October morning Freindlich put a pillow over his wife's face and pressed it tight until she quit breathing. He then tossed the pillow aside and wrenched apart the soldered light. When he heard the hiss of the gas, he hurriedly left the room, closing the door sharply behind him, leaving his dead wife lying beside the baby son she'd brought to bed with her. As the police pieced it together, he then walked out of the apartment, not trying to save the baby or any of the other children sleeping there.

But that tossed-aside pillow had dropped right on top of the sleeping infant. The little boy abruptly woke and began crying, struggling to get free. The Freindlichs' oldest child, a ten-year-old boy, heard his baby brother wailing and ran in to see what was wrong. He tried to shake his mother awake. But she didn't respond, no matter how hard he shook her. Now sobbing, he grabbed the baby and ran to the apartment next door. The neighbor grabbed a candle and hurried to check the darkened apartment. When she saw the dead woman in the bed, she ran to the grocer's place downstairs to call the police.

At first it looked like just another accident, maybe a suicide. Leah had been a sweet woman, the neighbors told the police, but worn down, just tired out. But something about the neighbor's story bothered the beat cops. If there was a lethal amount of illuminating gas in a room, it almost always ignited in the presence of fire, thanks to its explosive mixture of carbon monoxide and hydrogen. Apartments in the city blew up on a semiregular basis when someone unwittingly struck a match in a gas-filled room; Norris's office kept a file full of pictures showing blackened walls and fragmented furniture.

If illuminating gas had poisoned Leah Freindlich, it would have built up in the apartment. The room should have flashed to fire when the Good Samaritan ran in with her candle.

Back at the Bellevue morgue, the pathologist found the scenario equally dubious. The dead woman was sheet pale, all wrong for carbon monoxide poisoning, which tended to flush the skin pink. Before beginning an autopsy, he drew blood samples from her body and asked for a quick analysis from Gettler's laboratory. The lab results showed that the blood was loaded with carbon dioxide, the typical finding in suffocation, but there was no evidence of carbon monoxide. When the pathologist looked more closely at the body, hidden in the hair at the back of her neck he found a black bruising of fingerprints where someone had pressed fiercely against her skin.

Freindlich broke into sobs when he was arrested and begged the police to take him to the roof so that he could throw himself off. He couldn't have killed his wife, he said — no one could have wished her harm. He couldn't go to jail; what would happen to his children?

He wanted his old life back.

Carbon monoxide can be considered as a kind of chemical thug. It suffocates its victims simply by muscling oxygen out of the way.

In humans and many other animals, oxygen is transported in the bloodstream by the protein hemoglobin. Hemoglobin is classed as a metalloprotein because it contains the metal iron. Its structure, known as a heme, resembles a bright cluster of protein balls around a darker iron core. The iron in hemoglobin stains red blood cells, giving them that deep crimson color even as the protein itself efficiently moves oxygen through the body.

When a person inhales oxygen, the gas diffuses out of the lungs and into the bloodstream. Then because oxygen molecules are so attracted to iron, they bond to the hemoglobin. The result is called oxyhemoglobin, and in that neat package, the life-

sustaining gas is delivered to cells throughout the body. It seems a beautifully designed
system. But a chemical vulnerability is built
into it, which becomes very apparent with
exposure to a poison such as cyanide or
carbon monoxide. Both poisons attach to
hemoglobin far more effectively than oxygen.

Thus, these two chemical compounds are
life-threatening because they are opportunistic, making deft use of the body's essential metabolic systems. The attraction
between hemoglobin and carbon monoxide
is some two hundred times stronger than
that between hemoglobin and oxygen. No
wonder that CO — as an invading gas —
can cram into the blood cells, its tighter grip
allowing it to displace the looser oxygen
bonds. Oxyhemoglobin disappears; the
blood becomes saturated instead with carboxyhemoglobin, crowding oxygen from the
blood, locking it out of cells. The result is a
chemical suffocation.

The early symptoms of acute CO poisoning are drowsiness, headaches, dizziness,
confusion, and occasional nausea. In the
alcohol-hazed 1920s doctors tended to
mistake CO poisoning for drunkenness, according to records kept by Norris's office.
Sometimes the physicians just dismissed

signs of CO poisoning as the common mental illness seen among the city's derelicts. That wasn't necessarily surprising either. Exposure to carbon monoxide can also induce dementia, memory loss, irritability, a staggering loss of coordination, slurred speech, and even a deep feeling of depression.

Physicians so often got it wrong, at least in 1926, that a CO poisoning was often recognized just at the point when it was too late to save the victim. Or after the patient had been sent to the morgue.

There at Bellevue, in that sanctum of the dead, it took only a few simple tests to reveal a carbon monoxide death — or the absence of one, in the case of Leah Freindlich.

As CO absorbs into cells, it turns arterial blood from its normal dark bluish-red into a bright cherry color. The bright blood pinkens the skin at the same time, flushing it a deep rose color, sometimes mottled with red spotting. That was why Leah Freindlich's pallor alerted the pathologist on duty — he knew it contradicted the scene set by her husband.

On autopsy, following a carbon monoxide death, the muscle tissues gleam with crimson; so do the organs. The membranes of the throat and lungs are bright red, often covered by a weirdly frothy mucus layer. The brain can appear battered — swollen, dripping with bloody fluid. The cortex can be softened and blood-streaked. Some toxicologists argue that CO ultimately kills by damaging nervous system tissue until the lungs themselves are paralyzed.

In Alexander Gettler's laboratory, one of the simplest ways to test for CO was to extract blood from the corpse, pour some of it into a porcelain dish, and stir in some lye. Lye (a compound of sodium, hydrogen, and oxygen also known as caustic soda) turns normal blood into a dark, gelatinous ooze that, when held to the light, shows murky layers of greenish brown. But blood saturated with carbon monoxide doesn't darken that way; it stays an eerie, after-death crimson even as it jells, resembling glossy reddish aspic set into the white dish. In every chemical test, though, no matter what combination of materials is mixed into the blood, the dark/bright distinction persists. Blood containing oxyhemoglobin thickens to black, dark brown, or gray. Blood containing carboxyhemoglobin remains, as they say, blood red.

Chemists weren't sure exactly what produced that contrast, but they suspected it had something to do with the relentless grip that carbon monoxide exerts on iron components in hemoglobin. The strength of that connection, scientists speculated, might prevent the hemoglobin from breaking down so quickly, thus enabling it to keep staining the blood cells iron-red. But the looser bonds with oxygen might, instead, allow a decomposition of the iron, essentially causing a kind of tarnishing effect, in the way of any oxidized metal, darkening the blood as it did so.

That explanation was mostly educated guesswork, but of this one thing Gettler and his fellow toxicologists were certain: carbon monoxide did not like to let go of hemoglobin. Left for weeks during time tests, residing in stoppered bottles on the wooden counters of Gettler's lab, solutions containing carboxyhemoglobin would glow like the crimson hourglass on the abdomen of a black widow spider, like the clear carmine red of warning lights signaling danger to those who got too close.

When Charles Norris started as medical examiner, he'd decided to track every accidental illuminating gas death that occurred on his watch. During his first month in office — January 1918 — there were sixty-five such fatalities, an average of two a day.

The details of those deaths made it obvious that carbon monoxide does not discriminate in its victims. In the right circumstances, it will kill anyone. A newly married couple in an elegant brownstone just off Fifth Avenue on the Upper East Side were killed by gas escaping from a defective rubber hose; a woman living in midtown Manhattan was killed by gas escaping from tubing leading to a stove; a man on the Lower East Side was poisoned by gas escaping from a radiator; a man on the Upper West Side fell into bed drunk and failed to notice that the flame had blown out on two gas jets that fed the lamps in his room; a city inspector was killed by illuminating gas while inspecting the water meter in a basement; a man on Morningside Avenue, on the Upper West Side, was killed by gas escaping from a small gas heater in the bathroom.

In 1925 the details were of the same order, but the number of fatalities had gone up.

That January fifteen people were killed by gas in one terrible day. Among them — a man in Yonkers, killed by gas escaping from an unlighted burner on a stove; a baby, dead when his mother placed him by a poorly fitted stove for warmth; a Long Island man, killed by a leaky furnace; a Bronx man, his wife, and a guest staying in their apartment, dead due to another unlighted stove burner; a young mother and her baby, killed in Brooklyn by a faulty gas heater.

The U.S. Bureau of Mines, which had been investigating carbon monoxide risks in coal mines, released a report in the summer of 1926 stating that "the public generally does not appreciate the danger from gas leaks." The government was also weary of people reporting that a trained killer had set off a bomb when in actuality someone had merely left a gas jet open and then lit a cigarette. The bureau wanted to reassure the country's citizens that not every residential explosion was the work of the Black Hand Society.

It was usually the result of common carelessness.

The Black Hand — *La Mana Nera* in Italian — was an extortion syndicate organized by immigrants in New York and elsewhere (Chicago, San Francisco, and New Orleans) that used a simple and successful formula to acquire money. A letter was sent to a given target (often another Italian-American) threatening murder, arson, or kidnapping, sometimes all three, unless the society was paid off. The syndicate thrived by making good on its threats. It also believed in theatrical demonstrations, such as blowing up a car or apartment, shredding both property and victim into pieces. As its reputation for terror grew, the letters needed only the most basic signature — a hand printed in black ink.

In New York the Black Handers were mostly former Sicilians, headquartered in the neighborhood of Little Italy. One of the society's leaders, nicknamed Lupo (the Wolf), was so feared by other immigrants that they routinely crossed themselves at the mention of his name. The Wolf's favorite way to kill was to strangle a victim and then set the body on fire, preferably in a park for public viewing. Lupo and his colleagues did their best work in the early twentieth century, killing even police officers who interfered with their work. In 1909 the syndicate murdered a Manhattan police lieutenant in charge of the city's Italian Squad, which had been created as a response to organized crime. The lieutenant's funeral drew 250,000 mourners, a testament not only to how much he was admired but to how much the society was hated.

By the mid-1920s the Black Hand's tactics had mostly fallen out of fashion. The newer crime bosses felt that the extortion ring attracted too much attention; furthermore, the profits from bootlegging made blackmail schemes unnecessary. (The federal government estimated liquor syndicate profits at $3 billion in 1926.) But its name was still invoked to terrorize the disobedient. Thus the reaction to explosions that the government found so irritating. "Many disastrous explosions in buildings that are attributed to the Black Hand bombs or other mysteriously placed explosives are found on investigation to be caused by gas accumulations from leaks or burners that have become extinguished by drafts," the bureau noted stiffly.

The government suggested that the greater risk was the silent, far-too-pervasive leaking of illuminating gas into people's homes. In New York City alone deaths from illuminating gas continued to rise: 519 accidental asphyxiations reported in 1924 and 607 in the following year.

The Black Hand, at the height of its power, had never killed so many in one year.

The Leah Freindlich case posed a fascinating question for Gettler, at least the kind of question that obsessive forensic toxicologists find fascinating: could carbon monoxide be absorbed after death?

Leah Freindlich's blood had contained no meaningful carboxyhemoglobin, proving that the illuminating gas hadn't killed her. But what if the baby hadn't cried? What if the neighbor hadn't hurried to help, or the police had been slower to arrive? What if her body had had a few more hours to steep in the gas? Given more time, would the evidence have been blurred as the gas crept into the body?

There were a few tentative reports concerning such questions. For example, in a 1909 experiment a German researcher had exposed four stillborn babies to carbon monoxide for a full day. He reported that he saw signs of the gas in the lungs but nothing in the blood, not even in the heart. His conclusion was that if the gas were absorbed after death, it was only in bare trace amounts. Gettler thought the German scientist might be onto something. He just wished the study had been more meticulous. The researcher had merely recorded his observation of cherry-red color in lung tissue. He hadn't run tests for carboxyhemoglobin; he hadn't analyzed blood samples;

he hadn't produced the kind of enduring results that could be considered valid some fifteen years later.

Alexander Gettler wanted solid numbers, real data, as close to certainty as he could get. If the experiment he wanted didn't exist, he would just create it himself.

He started with a small collection of dead cats, collected from a city animal shelter. He then methodically exposed the bodies to carbon monoxide, putting them one at a time into a metal box, piping in illuminating gas through a small hole, sealing the box, and letting the cat corpses remain in that CO-soaked environment for one to five days. Gettler then drew blood from the animals, from locations around the body, including the heart.

He was looking for that familiar bright discoloration in the blood, for the chemical signature of carboxyhemoglobin. First, though, he would have to adjust for an environmental complication: exposure to city air.

Thanks to the streets overflowing with automobiles, the increasing reliance on gas appliances, and the sprouting of industrial factories along urban corridors, every living creature, especially in the big cities, now inhaled a constant dose of carbon monoxide.

Animal studies conducted in New York showed that dogs and cats, for instance, had a predictable amount of carboxyhemoglobin saturating their blood. The average saturation in rural areas was less than one percent; but in New York City, CO levels in household pets and feral cats, like those in Gettler's study, ran 1.5 percent or higher.

Even after five days of concentrated CO exposure, however, Gettler's dead cats remained at a basic urban blood level. That result suggested that the gas did not permeate their bodies after death. It seemed probable that the same would be true in people. To be sure, he needed to conduct similar experiments on dead human beings.

This was where working in a medical examiner's office offered an important advantage; dead bodies were the routine of each working day. Most of the corpses that came to the morgue had families, friends, or lovers who claimed them. But others seemed to belong to no one. They were the unwanted children — the baby who had been found stuffed into a Gladstone bag and left on an Upper West Side sidewalk — the floaters from the East River, the bums from the Bowery who drank a lethal dose of

Smoke and turned up tumbled along the brick wall of an alley. Their bodies ended up in Potter's Field, the city burial ground for the John and Jane Does of the morgue, the unknowns, the lost, the bodies left unclaimed because their families couldn't afford to give them a burial.

The city and the state now had so many alcohol-poisoned dead that one New York assemblyman compared Prohibition enforcers to the Borgia family. "The government," he warned, "is surpassing the Italian fiends of the Middle Ages by dealing death to its own people, who constitute the backbone of the Republic." There were so many corpses that the city could hardly keep up with burying them. In the midst of that overload, Norris decided to let Gettler experiment on three of the Bowery dead, currently residing in the refrigerated drawers of the morgue's storage room, destined for unmarked pauper's graves.

To do the experiment, Gettler had a larger metal box built: six feet long, two and half feet wide, and two feet deep. The tightly fitted lid had a rubber gasket set in place where a tube could be inserted to pipe in carbon monoxide. Each end of the box was fitted with a stopcock. Each time "the body was placed in the box and the lid was fastened tightly," Gettler wrote, "illuminating gas was passed through the box for thirty minutes and the stopcocks then closed."

He left the first two dead men in the box for twenty-four hours, the third for forty-two hours. In all three cases, just as with the cats, the blood in the dead men's hearts remained at normal urban levels. Soaking in carbon monoxide for hours after death had had no effect at all. Death created its own bleak protective shield; without breath, carbon monoxide was just another gas aimlessly swirling in the air.

In October 1926 Norris issued his yearly analysis of deaths in New York City. He'd instituted that procedure when taking office. Insurance companies around the country now requested the report.

This one confirmed that automobiles and their often-drunken drivers remained the city's greatest killers, taking 1,272 lives in a year. There had also been 984 suicides (almost 400 by illuminating gas), 356 murders (mostly shootings), and 585 alcohol-related deaths. There was also the elevator problem: 87 people had died in elevator accidents during the year — 47 falls into open shafts, 36 crushed by the doors, three killed when cables broke and the machines fell.

Then six people had been killed playing baseball, six people had died in sleighing accidents, football had killed one, three had died in fistfights, and eight people had lost their lives in diving accidents. The list could go on and on — and did. The medical examiner's office counted a total of 5,581 deaths from such nonnatural causes that year, which — as Norris also noted — was pretty average for the city.

The gloomy statistics led the way into a chilly December, clouded by fog. The mist lapped along the rivers and muffled the harbors; stranded vessels in low-floating clouds gave an eerie unreality to the usual creak of boats rubbing against docks in the water. Footsteps thudded unexpectedly in the mist; people startled at the most ordinary sound.

In the first week of that foggy month, far too early in the morning, a Brooklyn police officer patrolling along the East River saw a man moving stealthily toward a poorly lit part of the wharf where freight-bearing ships from India docked. There was a full moon and the wind was shuffling the mist. The officer could see that the man was bent slightly, carrying a heavy-looking bundle, as he approached the India Wharf.

Curious, the patrolman edged closer. The man placed his burden on the edge of the pier. Officer James Anderson shouted for him to stand still. He wanted to look at the bundle. But the man instead kicked the object into the river and fled into the mist. Anderson shouted again, and then pulled out his revolver and fired it three times into the air.

Another patrolman, hearing the shots, came running and almost collided with the fugitive, tackling him to the ground. What was that package? the police asked. Who are you? What are you doing here? The man looked like a workman, dressed in corduroy pants, a heavy pea jacket, and a cap pulled down over his forehead. He was dark, short, and silent. He shook his head, refusing to answer.

The policemen's voices became louder, repeating the questions. The man still shook his head, glaring back at them. The rumble of a car's engine drawing closer made them all jump. It was a battered black taxi, and the driver, on his way home, had seen the chase. He could at least identify the man in the pea jacket as his neighbor. Both lived in a cluster of apartments on Sackett Street in

Brooklyn. The man being questioned was a longshoreman named Francesco Travia.

Even through the shadows, the cops thought Travia looked ill, oddly flushed, his face rimed with black stubble. He folded his arms tighter. He wouldn't tell them what was in the bundle, now vanished into the river. He wouldn't tell them why he was there on the India Wharf. They took him back to the Hamilton Street police station and studied him in the light. The bottoms of his gray trousers were smudged dark red. Take off your shoes, they said. His socks were sodden with blood.

The officers locked him into a cell and went directly to his apartment. It was what people sometimes called a bloody shambles. On the kitchen floor was a dead woman. Or rather half a dead woman. The upper part of the body — torso, arms, battered head — lay between the table and the stove in a clotted pool of red. A spattered butcher's knife and a chisel sat on a table, smeared and streaked with gore.

The officers returned hastily to their precinct station and formally arrested Travia on murder and dismemberment charges. A day later the medical examiner's office, Charles Norris and Alexander Gettler working in tandem, would prove the police wrong.

The office was short-staffed that night, so Charles Norris was on call. He made his usual entrance, even at three in the morning, stepping out of his chauffeur-driven automobile, dressed against the cold in dark overcoat and fedora. He followed the policemen up the wooden stairs to Travia's apartment, laid his outer garments on a chair, and walked over to inspect the dismembered corpse.

His thick eyebrows drew together in a familiar frown. The blood pooled around the half-body was a bright cherry red. He bent to look closer at the woman's face. It was flushed pink, even following this horrible death. Norris's reaction was recorded by a crime writer and would later become part of his often theatrical legend. He walked over to the waiting detectives and announced, "Boys, you can't hold this man for murder."

The Brooklyn police assured him that they could.

The body was taken to the Bellevue morgue. It had barely arrived when the cops at the Hamilton Street station called to say they were sending a man and his daughter down to look at the body. The sixteen-year-old daughter had come to the police station to report her mother missing. The girl's description — a stocky woman in her early forties with dark hair, heavy brows above brown eyes, a round face, and a thick neck — matched their corpse perfectly.

It took Alice Fredericksen and her father, Frederick, a while to get to Bellevue by train and surface car. In the interim the morgue attendants did their best to disguise the damage, heaping sheets over the corpse until only the face was visible. When Fredericksen arrived, he took one shrinking look and identified his wife, Anna, lying on the marble table.

On further inquiry, it turned out that the Fredericksens knew the murder suspect. Their family ran a rooming house on Henry Street, around the corner from his apartment building. Travia was a loner and a drinker, but no one had thought of him as a violent man. And Anna had been plain easygoing, not the kind of woman to provoke a murder. Both father and daughter were shocked — and bewildered.

In his quiet laboratory, Gettler took blood from Anna Fredericksen's heart and began putting it through the standard chemical tests. In each glass vessel, each ceramic dish, the bloody solutions, instead of turning the darkish grays of normal oxygenated blood, flamed that brilliant red. Her blood was saturated with carboxyhemoglobin. And as corpses didn't absorb the gas, and as the saturation level was lethal, Anna Fredericksen had been dead, Gettler reported, before Travia had picked up his knife.

Francesco Travia had come to New York with his children twenty-two years earlier, after his wife died in Italy. His parents had immigrated before him; they still lived in Coney Island. Once in New York, he'd decided on a new and solitary life. He took to calling himself Frank, left his children with his parents, found a job, and stayed alone in his little apartment. He preferred to drink alone as well, spending his Saturday nights with a pint of whatever bootleg whiskey was available.

As he told investigators — in a sudden, frightened confession — Anna Fredericksen had come by in search of some booze. They were out of alcohol at home, she complained. She was known as a heavy drinker in the neighborhood. Her husband admitted to police that she "frequently drank intoxicants" and that her usual bootlegger had been unable to deliver that weekend.

Travia said that he and Anna had finished his own supply of liquor, sitting at his kitchen table. When he tried to get her to leave, they'd fallen into an argument, and then, well, he'd felt incredibly sleepy and had fallen asleep at the table. He woke sometime later, he wasn't sure, foggy-headed. She was still there, lying on the floor. He went to shake her awake. She was creepily cold to the touch, creepily stiff. He could only think, he told police, that he must have killed her while they'd argued, shaken her to death, strangled her, he didn't know. But he did know there was a dead woman on the floor. And, he was absolutely sure that he'd be charged with murder once she was found.

So there in the dark of early morning, he decided that his only chance was to get rid of the body. But she was a big woman, tall and chunky, too large to simply haul away over a shoulder. Maybe the alcohol had confused him, he admitted, or maybe it was something else. But Travia decided that he'd have to cut her into smaller pieces and then get rid of her one part at a time.

He used his butcher knife to do the sawing and his chisel to splinter through the bones. Then he wrapped the lower half of her body in newspapers, burlap bags, and an old raincoat and carried it down to the river. He hadn't figured out what to do with the upper half, but then he never got that chance. That was his story. He swore it was true. And whether one believed it depended on whether one believed in the scientific results from Bellevue.

Norris could talk all he wanted about the significance of pink faces; Gettler could discuss carboxyhemoglobin until he grew hoarse. But in Brooklyn the police found bloody knives and body parts more convincing.

Which meant that Francesco Travia was, after all, arraigned to stand trial on murder. And as Charles Norris saw it, the New York City medical examiner's office would have a date in court, a chance to prove very publicly that scientific evidence was a tangible thing, as real, as convincing — and as influential — as any other evidence presented in a courtroom.

Some months later, in March 1927, a Kings County jury acquitted Frank Travia of murder. Norris had predicted that the gruesome nature of the case would make sure people paid attention. In fact, publicity surrounding his case had gained Travia an unusually well-connected young lawyer,

Alfred E. Smith Jr., son of the governor of New York.

It was Smith Jr.'s first case, and it went perfectly for him. Unlike the police, he'd found the medical evidence very impressive, enough so that he built his whole case around it. Smith's witness list was short: the building owner, to say that he'd discovered that a coffeepot on Travia's stove had boiled over, putting out the burner flame, allowing gas to drift through the apartment; Alexander O. Gettler, to testify that carbon monoxide poisoning had caused the woman's death; and Frank Travia, to describe his panicked reaction on finding her dead.

Travia was found not guilty of murder but guilty of illegally dismembering a dead body. The difference was enormous; it meant that he went to prison instead of the electric chair. When the trial concluded, Travia's attorney returned home and found a telegram from Albany waiting for him. The governor wanted to congratulate him on his debut as a criminal lawyer, on proving that the cause of death was not a drunken Italian laborer but an all-too-common, all-too-lethal household gas.

The governor did not also congratulate the scientists of the medical examiner's office, but they celebrated anyway. All that patient chemistry, all Gettler's time-consuming experiments with carbon monoxide, had helped save a man from the electric chair, despite the doubts expressed by the police. As much as Norris's lectures at the police academy, as much as those scheduled tours of Gettler's laboratory, the Travia case illustrated that forensic toxicology was a powerful — and credible — tool.

The days when chemists killed cats in courtrooms, and medical experts waved chloroform vials in front of nervous jurors, were demonstrably over. They could make their points with sober testimony and charts of chemical analysis. They hadn't entirely figured out carbon monoxide, true, and no one was sure how to contain the environmental hazards posed by the gas. But Norris and Gettler had saved one life this day, and they were confident that they could save others.

Call it a coming-of-age party for forensic toxicology — there in the third-floor laboratory at Bellevue the bubble and hiss of beakers sounded like victory music in the air around them.

# SEVEN:
## METHYL ALCOHOL
## $(CH_3OH)$
### 1927

---

The rumors began in the summer of 1926. Government chemists were developing a secret project in the aid of Prohibition, people whispered. Dry officials issued warnings that drinking was about to become more risky. The Great War had taught people that chemists could be more dangerous than other scientists. A new chemists' war was brewing, it was said, pitting government scientists against those employed by the country's powerful bootlegging empires.

It was no secret that the federal government seethed with frustration over the flouting of anti-alcohol laws. When Prohibition went into effect, backed by a Constitutional amendment no less, its supporters had assumed citizens would, however reluctantly, obey the law. The succeeding years had proved them wrong. Many now drank more than ever, more recklessly, more adventurously. In Washington, D.C., where the Volstead Act — which provided for enforcement of the Eighteenth Amendment — had been militantly approved, the police reported nearly a ten-fold increase in drunk driving arrests since the legislation was enacted.

The illegal alcohol trade had not only flourished but grown more sophisticated. In the mid-1920s much of the available spirits came from stolen industrial alcohol, which was famously poisonous. Since 1906 the U.S. government had required that manufacturers denature (poison) industrial alcohol or else pay liquor taxes. By the 1920s some seventy denaturing formulas existed. The simplest formulas just added extra methyl, or wood, alcohol into the mix. Others mixed a cocktail of bitter-tasting but less lethal compounds, designed to make the alcohol taste so awful that it became undrinkable.

With the use of such tainted supplies the liquor syndicates needed chemists to help them clean up industrial alcohol. By paying well enough, the bootleggers secured some very able scientists. The chemists had quickly neutralized the simplest of the denaturing additives. Formula 39b, used in production of alcohol for perfume and cosmetics, was a favorite of the illegal alcohol trade because it was not particularly dangerous and thus "renatured" nicely. The heavy-duty industrial versions were deadlier and more difficult to make safe. But recently the bootleggers' chemists claimed to have found a way to renature even the most lethal versions. They'd found — or so they claimed — a process that caused the methyl alcohol to precipitate to the bottom of a container where it could mostly be filtered out. The resulting spirits were more poisonous than traditional grain alcohol but not so much that the consumers dropped dead in the street.

Amid indications that the bootlegger chemists were gaining on the denaturing front, dry advocates in Congress demanded tougher measures and better poisons. Their position was that if Americans persisted in flouting the law, if they continued to evade the hardworking law enforcement agents, then perhaps the best way to enforce Prohibition was to make alcohol so deadly that even the sellout chemists working for the crime syndicates couldn't rescue it. If alcohol was truly undrinkable, the argument went, even the most devoted boozer would have to give it up.

And those summer 1926 rumors? They were absolutely true. The government was experimenting with new denaturing agents, planning to require much greater amounts of methyl alcohol in the denaturing process. Other poisons were under review as well, including benzene, kerosene, and brucine (a plant alkaloid closely related to strychnine). Federal chemists defended this practice as simple law enforcement: "ignorance, politics and bootlegging" were the real problem, according to a report by the American Chemical Society, which complained that "the continual controversy for and against Prohibition and over the methods for the enforcement" of the law was starting to create public hostility against hardworking scientists.

By 1926 federal chemists had devised ten new formulas dedicated to deterring bootleggers and their customers. But the black market chemists proved able in countering these moves. In the spring, formula number six, which included mercury bichloride, was overcome. In September, numbers three and four had to be discarded. Formulas one and five — which contained the most methyl alcohol (plus some benzene and pyridine) — remained dangerous, but that was mostly because, as one government chemist told reporters, no one had ever figured out how to completely detoxify wood alcohol.

It was hard to miss the conclusion. Prohibition chemists didn't have to create exotic formulas. Wood alcohol, methyl alcohol, whatever you chose to call it, was still the best poison at hand.

As the year pulled toward its close, on a festively lit Christmas Eve, a man came running — make that weaving — into Bellevue's emergency room, claiming that Santa Claus had chased him from Fifth Avenue with a baseball bat. He was among the sixty-five people who came to the hospital in two days, all sickened by holiday celebrations.

The problem, Charles Norris reported, was primarily poisoned liquor. The latest round of hooch available in the city had not cleaned up well. It remained an unusually nasty soup of government-added impurities and methyl alcohol. Eight people died at Bellevue, and fifteen others were admitted. Two days after Christmas twenty-three were dead and eighty-nine hospitalized. Most of them later were packed into the alcoholic ward at Bellevue, hallucinating, vomiting, blinded by wood alcohol, bundled onto cots like so many sticks of kindling.

On December 28 a furious Norris issued a public statement:

The government knows it is not stopping drinking by putting poison in alcohol. It knows what the bootleggers are doing with it and yet it continues its poisoning processes, heedless of the fact that people determined to drink are daily absorbing that poison. Knowing this to be true, the United States Government must be charged with the moral responsibility for the deaths that poisoned liquor causes, although it cannot be held legally responsible.

The equally furious response came from Wayne Wheeler, general counsel of the Anti-Saloon League of America. He accused Norris, and the newspapers that had quoted the medical examiner, of being in league with bootleggers. The fact was that these so-called victims had violated the law, Wheeler said, and deserved no sympathy for their illegal, and also idiotic, behavior.

A speakeasy patron was "in the same category as the man who walks into a drug store, buys a bottle of carbolic acid with a label on it marked 'poisonous,' and drinks the contents," Wheeler asserted. If these individuals chose to engage in suicidal actions, he added, that was their choice and no reason to change an important and righteous national policy.

It became obvious on the next day, the last day of 1926, that Wheeler's position was also the federal government's position. The Treasury Department announced that it had decided to require that denatured alcohol be more poisonous. The amount of methyl alcohol in all formulas would be doubled at a minimum. Mostly that meant going from the traditional 2 percent to 4 percent of contents. But if that didn't serve, then the Prohibition chemists had developed a Special Formula One, which called for 5 to 10 percent methyl alcohol.

The chances of bootleggers distilling that out were slim; some stills might actually concentrate the poison. But as Wheeler had made so clear, that was the drinker's problem.

The president of Columbia University was fed up with all of it.

Nicholas Murray Butler had opposed the Eighteenth Amendment from the start. He didn't oppose regulation of saloons, but doing so by constitutional amendment, he said, was overkill. And by 1927, seven years into the social experiment, any idiot could see that Prohibition had been an enormous mistake, Butler said, one that could be

271

remedied only by replacing the country's leaders.

Butler announced in February that he would himself run for president, seeking to become the Republican Party candidate on an anti-Prohibition platform, which would call for repealing the Eighteenth Amendment and returning the power to regulate alcohol to the individual states. Butler's declaration, though, received less attention than the vituperative answers it generated.

"The people of the United States will never make Uncle Sam a bartender," Wheeler responded. Nor would they ever elect someone like Butler, a man "soaked in avarice and rum." Law-abiding dry advocates represented the majority of Americans, Wheeler added. They would always reject being led by a representative of New York City, a den of "bootleggers, rum-runners, owners of speakeasy property, wet newspapers, underworld denizens, alcoholic slaves and personal liberty fanatics . . . Neither Nicholas Murray Butler nor any other apologist for the liquor crowd will ever occupy the White House."

Butler, in his public response to Wheeler, sounded amused, maybe a little bored: "It sounds as if something had happened to trouble him." But Wheeler and his allies —

for the moment, at least — still wielded real political power. Butler did not gain the presidential nomination — it went to Secretary of Commerce Herbert Hoover, who promised continued economic prosperity and endorsed Prohibition as an "experiment noble in purpose."

Much later Hoover's friends would reveal that the experiment had been a little too noble for Hoover, who regularly stopped by the Belgian embassy on his way home from Commerce. Since the embassy was technically on foreign soil, he could drink there legally and be guaranteed some very good-quality alcohol as well.

The pathologists and chemists of the New York City medical examiner's office viewed the government's deliberate poisoning of alcohol as an act of betrayal. Handling an average of twelve thousand bodies a year, they were accustomed to unnecessary loss of life — nearly half of those corpses were the result of accident, suicide, or murder.

But they weren't accustomed to having their national government adopt a policy known to kill people in droves. In the offices at Bellevue, their outrage crackled like a current in the air.

In January the usually reserved Gettler

marched off to meet with the New York press, bearing pages of information on lives taken by poisoned alcohol. As always, Gettler said, money bought greater safety. The well-heeled clubbers, the wealthy lovers of jazz-flavored cocktails, could afford the pricey higher-quality alcohol on the market. Many of them routinely invited their bootleggers to parties, gaining some personal insurance against poisoning. But the poor could buy only the alcoholic dregs: nickel whiskey from the tenement stills, the Smoke cocktails of the Bowery, straight wood alcohol. More than anyone else, the city's impoverished residents were paying the real price of Prohibition.

The statistics that Gettler delivered to city newspapers bore this out: in the year 1926 alone some twelve hundred in New York City had been sickened or blinded or both by drinking some form of industrial alcohol; another four hundred people had died, most of them from Manhattan's Lower East Side, Gas House district, Hell's Kitchen, and like neighborhoods in the other boroughs. "The figures exceed the number who died from alcoholism in the days of the saloon," he said, his sentences dry and cold with determination. "It is impossible to estimate the effect which this poisoned liquor has had on the nervous systems of those taking it and who are not made ill enough to be brought to the hospital for treatment. It is clear enough, however, that the liquor which contains enough poison to kill so many is slowly but surely killing many others."

Mayor Jimmy Walker's first response was that of any dedicated drinking man: "If I had a club I would hit on the head myself any man who sold poison liquor and I would not wait for a policeman." His second was that of a mayor confronted with a public health crisis: he wanted a report. He wanted his chief medical examiner to give him a tally and evaluation of alcohol deaths in the city.

Charles Norris was never a man to miss a moment of opportunity.

His reply to Walker's request, published in February, started small, using Bellevue Hospital as a case study. At the start of Prohibition doctors there had treated about a dozen cases of moonshine and wood alcohol poisoning every year. Maybe a fourth of them had been fatal. But in 1926 the hospital had treated 716 people for alcoholic hallucinations, blindness, and even paralysis due to poisoned alcohol. Sixty-one of those patients had died. And that figure didn't include deaths due to chronic alcoholism — those had numbered 87 in 1918. In the current year of 1927, Norris predicted, based on January and February deaths, more than 700 city residents would drink themselves to death by year's end. (He would be proved right.)

Not only were people drinking more under Prohibition, he said, but with full government complicity they were imbibing alcohol that hardly deserved the name. He and his staff had analyzed bottles from speakeasies and Smoke joints, from hip flasks found in the pockets of bodies on the street. Every drink contained methyl alcohol but they also found gasoline, benzene, cadmium, iodine, zinc, mercury salts, nicotine, ether, formaldehyde, chloroform, camphor, carbolic acid, quinine, and acetone. No wonder the newest nickname for the stuff coming from the tenement stills and grocery store moonshiners was "white mule": the clear liquid, it was said, left the drinker feeling kicked in the head.

"There is practically no pure whiskey available" anyplace in the city, Norris warned. "My opinion, based on actual experience of the medical examiner's staff and myself, is that there is actually no Prohibition. All the people who drank before Prohibition are drinking now — provided they are still alive."

The New York papers — those wet publications so despised by the Anti-Saloon League — promptly embraced Norris's report as evidence of a government policy gone haywire. "Prohibition in this area is a complete failure," the *Herald Tribune*'s editorial page declared, "enforcement a travesty, the public a victim of poisonous liquor." Columnist Heywood Broun wrote in the *New York World*, "The Eighteenth is the only amendment which carries the death penalty." And the *Evening World* described the federal government as a mass poisoner, noting that no administration had been more successful in "undermining the health of its own people."

The impact of Norris's report rippled outward beyond his city. U.S. Senator James Reed of Missouri told the *St. Louis Post* that the New York medical examiner had convinced him that Prohibition supporters were uncivilized: "Only one possessing the instincts of a wild beast would desire to kill or make blind the man who takes a drink of liquor, even if he purchased it from one violating the Prohibition statutes." The *St. Paul Pioneer Press* called the government "an accessory to murder when it uses deadly denaturants." Even the *Cleveland Plain Dealer,* which had supported the Eighteenth Amendment, said that sympathy for the cause did not mean "we wish to inflict punishment upon those who persist in violating Prohibition laws."

And the *Chicago Tribune* put it like this:

Normally, no American government would engage in such business. It would not and does not set a trap gun loaded with nails to catch a counterfeiter. It would not put "Rough on Rats" on a cheese sandwich even to catch a mail robber. It would not poison postage stamps to get a citizen known to be misusing the mails. It is only in the curious fanaticism of Prohibition that any means, however barbarous, are considered justified.

Dry newspapers found Norris less persuasive. Alcohol killed thousands of people long before Prohibition was enacted, they pointed out. "Must Uncle Sam guarantee safety first for souses?" asked Nebraska's *Omaha Bee.* The *Springfield Republican* of southern Illinois dismissed the whole outcry as "wet propaganda." And the *Pittsburgh*

*Gazette Times* pointedly raised a question that puzzled even opponents of the law: why would people persist in drinking white mule and Smoke, paint shop hooch and bathtub gin, when they must know that it could kill them?

Didn't the obstinate guzzler bear some responsibility? Wasn't it possible that "the drinker himself is to blame for the ills that befall him as a result of his libations?" the Pittsburgh editors wrote plaintively.

As the bodies piled up in the Bellevue morgue, Norris pondered that question himself. Why would anyone play Russian roulette with a glass of liquor? Why did people continue drinking the Borgia cocktails — as one politician called them — of Prohibition?

One reason, perhaps, was that speakeasy patrons didn't appreciate the risk. They didn't realize that the newest version of denatured alcohol was more dangerous than the wood-alcohol-laced whiskies they remembered, or the oldtime moonshine, smuggled over from Kentucky or Tennessee. The city's drinkers had no reason to trust government warnings; they believed that the anti-alcohol administration was deliberately exaggerating the risks. This was partly true, of course, but unfortunately not entirely.

In 1923 German chemists had figured out how to make a synthetic methyl alcohol called methanol. The key was to put carbon, oxygen, and hydrogen into an industrial pressure cooker and superheat the mixture to more than 400 degrees Fahrenheit. The result was a near-perfect methyl alcohol. Synthetic methanol was extraordinarily pure and extremely cheap to make; within a couple years the wood alcohol factories were closing their doors, giving way to the new chemistry. In 1925 Norris issued a warning that German methanol was being sold on the streets of Manhattan for half the price of the old wood alcohol. It wasn't hard to find, he added: "We use it in our automobile radiators and around the house in cleaning fluids, paints, insect sprays and beauty lotions. It is present in over two hundred articles of common household and industrial use."

He hoped people would understand, he'd said, that the word "pure," in this case, did not mean "safe." In the case of methanol, it meant purely "poisonous."

Methyl alcohol had another confounding factor. It wasn't one of those poisons, like cyanide, that could make one violently sick in a few minutes and kill in less than a quarter-hour. Drinking white mule didn't feel like swallowing poison. Not at all. It felt like sharing a friendly drink on a corner, in a basement bar, giving the familiar buzzing sense of intoxication.

If a drinker cared to notice, the first difference between methyl and grain (ethyl) alcohol was in how long the buzz lasted. With methyl alcohol, the period of cheerful inebriation was shorter; the sensation of a hangover could come within an hour or two. If the dose was high enough, a few drinks rapidly led to headache, dizziness, nausea, a staggering lack of coordination, confusion, and finally an overpowering need to sleep. When Norris called methanol pure poison, he wasn't exaggerating. The lethal undiluted dose was as little as two teaspoons for a child, perhaps a quarter cup for an adult man. That modest amount, far too often, was a direct path to blindness, followed by coma, followed by death.

Unlike the grain alcohol served before Prohibition, methyl (wood) alcohol is not easily broken down in the body. The enzymes in the liver that neatly dispatch ethyl alcohol struggle with methyl. As a result, the more poisonous version lingers in the system, simmers longer in the organs, and metabolizes away only slowly. And as it stews, it becomes more poisonous. The primary by-products of methyl alcohol in the human body, as chemists had discovered, are formaldehyde and formic acid.

Formaldehyde is a known irritant poison, capable of causing severe internal damage, and formic acid is equally destructive, best known to scientists as an essential part of the venom in bee stings. People poisoned by methyl alcohol would often seem to recover from that first bout of dizzy sickness, feel better while the alcohol was being metabolized, and then ten to thirty hours later be poisoned again by the breakdown products.

First, their vision would blur. The optic nerve and retina are acutely vulnerable to formic acid salts. The nerve, with its continual processing of images, runs in a high metabolic state, causing blood to circulate through it rapidly — which causes poison to be delivered there continuously. Autopsies often revealed a startling atrophy of the optic nerve area, the surrounding tissue swollen, bloody, and spongy. Methyl alcohol and its by-products caused similar damage in the parietal cortex, a region of the brain essential in processing vision. It concentrated as well in the hardworking lungs — the breakdown of pulmonary tissue was what usually killed people.

In an essay titled "Our Experiment in Extermination," published in the *North American Review,* Norris mounted an even more pointed attack on government policy, this time taking his case directly to a national audience and directly mocking Hoover's description of Prohibition as a "noble experiment."

Like Gettler, Norris was particularly outraged by the punishment that the anti-alcohol laws had visited upon the poor. The really poisonous liquor, he wrote, was sold in low dives, funneled from backroom stills, and delivered by bootleggers "who cannot afford expensive protection and deal in low grade stuff with a low grade of trade." Of those killed by methyl alcohol, "only a fraction . . . come from the upper levels of thirsty society." The protection offered to the wealthy, the powerful, the artists, and the politicians had helped give illegal alcohol a kind of high-life image, a dangerous seductive allure: "Prohibition has undoubtedly bred a glamour to surround alcohol . . . it permits the tanning and galvanizing of young stomachs and countenances young debauchery."

Norris wasn't opposed to cocktail parties or to members of the twenty-something set drinking in moderation. His concern was that new drinkers could no longer start lightly, beginning with a glass of wine or a friendly beer at the local pub. Everyone now had to start with the hard stuff because not much else was available. "Old and normal tastes for beer and wines must now be largely satisfied with deadlier intoxicants — doubly deadly intoxicants."

In early 1927, wet legislators in Congress tried to pass a law to halt the extra poisoning of industrial alcohol. They had failed, overwhelmed by dry legislators' declarations that no one would be dead if people simply obeyed the law and tried to live in a morally upright fashion. Norris, in response, argued that this imposition of one group's personal beliefs on the rest of society could not be justified as moral.

Further, he said, the experiment of the Eighteenth Amendment proved his point. Yes, the law had changed the old ways of life, the old style of drinking. But it had created another drinking lifestyle and another kind of immorality: "It has failed to reduce, moderate or control heavy drinking. It has created a new social order of bootleggers, and its blunders have protected an infant industry until it is now so secure in the law and the profits as to be a real menace to our national security and integrity.

"And," Norris concluded, "death follows at its heels."

That March a murder out on Long Island distracted the chief medical examiner, briefly at least, from his crusade against government alcohol policies. It was the kind of murder that would have distracted almost anyone.

It started with a dose of mercury bichloride, then a measure of chloroform. Several tumblers of alcohol followed, and then a lead sash weight to the man's head. It finished with picture wire pulled tight around the victim's neck. To such a rare case, the word *overkill* could be applied without hyperbole.

The complicated murder of Albert Snyder put the men of the medical examiner's office — especially Alexander Gettler — on public display. It rapidly became a very public event, the story of the spring for tabloid newspapers and their sensation-loving readers.

The plotting of Snyder's murder — by his charming wife, Ruth, and her doting boyfriend, Judd Gray, was so bizarre that the novelist James M. Cain would later use it as a basis for his two best-known novels, *The Postman Always Rings Twice* and *Double Indemnity*. It was the dark theme of betrayal that attracted him, Cain later explained. For others, the ridiculous side of the crime triumphed. The *New York American* columnist Damon Runyon once suggested that the murderers should have been convicted on the charge of being inept idiots.

And the killing itself, Runyon added, should have been called "The Dumb-Bell Murder."

In March 1927 Ruth and Albert Snyder had been married for twelve years. He was a forty-four-year-old art editor at Hearst's *Motor Boating* magazine. She was thirty-two, a pretty and playful blonde. They had a ten-year-old daughter, Lorraine, for which Albert had not forgiven his wife — he'd wanted a son.

In fact, Albert was almost never satisfied. He expected Ruth to keep a meticulous home. He criticized every misplaced dish or dirty corner in the house. He slapped both his wife and his daughter around when they annoyed him. And in the way of Prohibition, he was becoming a heavy drinker. He brewed his own beer in the basement, patronizing the local bootlegger when he wanted the hard stuff. It never seemed to occur to Snyder that he'd taught his wife to hate him, or perhaps he didn't care. Ruth escaped as much as possible, taking the train to Manhattan to lunch with friends while Lorraine was at school.

In the summer of 1925, at the lunch counter of a Fifth Avenue restaurant, she idly flirted with the man on the next stool over, a rather attractive businessman with curly dark hair and horn-rimmed glasses. By the end of that summer, Ruth Snyder was regularly meeting Judd Gray at the Waldorf-Astoria, the hotel he used while conducting business in the city. Gray was a corset salesman who lived in East Orange, New Jersey. His wife disliked the boozing he did while entertaining clients, so he had a good reason to stay in Manhattan while on business.

Two years into their affair, the lovers decided to run away together, but they needed money. Gray, better educated and more financially astute, helped Ruth to arrange $45,000 worth of life insurance for Albert. The policy carried a double indemnity clause. If his death was "due to misadventure," the payout would be $90,000.

Neither of them wanted to wait too long

for the money; they could start new lives only if Albert would cooperate.

On the morning of Sunday, March 20, 1927, Lorraine Snyder hysterically hammered on the next-door neighbor's kitchen door. She'd found her mother bound and unconscious on the living room floor. When help arrived, Ruth woke slowly. She whispered, painfully, that burglars had broken in, tied her up, and clubbed her on the head.

The neighbors ran down the hall, looking for her husband. When they pushed open the bedroom door, they found Albert Snyder lying facedown on a blood-streaked pillow. A length of picture wire was twisted around his neck, its ends sticking in the air.

When the police arrived, Ruth told them that she and her husband had gone to a bridge party the previous night, returning at about two in the morning. She'd hardly fallen asleep when she heard a noise in the hall. Rising to investigate, she saw an enormous man coming toward her, "an Italian-looking" thug. She'd prepared to scream, but then everything had gone dark. He must have cracked her on the head, she said, and she'd awakened hours later to find herself trussed on the floor.

The house was a shambles, sofa cushions

thrown on the living room floor, pots and pans scattered around the kitchen. The floor surrounding the bed where Albert Snyder lay dead was in a similar state. But strangely enough, or so the detectives thought, the clutter in the bedroom included Albert's shining gold pocket watch, with its pricey platinum chain.

From that puzzling point on, the story proceeded to fall apart.

The doctor examining Ruth Snyder found no head injury, no bump, no bruise, nothing to account for what she insisted had been six hours of unconsciousness. She'd been discovered with her feet bound, but her hands had not been tied. Why, wondered the detectives, hadn't she just untied her feet? Ruth insisted that, although her husband's watch remained, some of her own jewelry and furs were definitely missing. But the three rings and silver bar pin turned up, wrapped in a rag and stuffed under her mattress, and the police found her squirrel coat in a trunk in the basement.

Also in the basement, they found something more damning. In a corner where Albert Snyder had made a workshop, they discovered a toolbox pushed under a bench. Inside, along with screwdrivers and hammers, was an iron sash weight, smeared with blood. The rounded edges of the weight matched perfectly the rounded bruises they'd found around Snyder's face.

The following morning Ruth Snyder confessed.

That is, she blamed Judd Gray for everything. He'd worked out the life insurance business. He'd bought the murder weapons. He'd come to the house shortly after she and her husband returned from the bridge party. He had a key to her home; she had seen him standing in a shadowed corner. He was wearing rubber gloves. "My God, Judd," she'd gasped. "You're not going to do that, are you?" But he was determined, she said. He'd made her do it.

A police hunt for Judd Gray found him on a northbound train out of the city. He was carrying a bottle of poisoned whiskey — one that Ruth Snyder had asked him to bring, he said. She was the killer, Gray assured the police, who'd poisoned her husband and slugged him to death with a sash weight.

The bungled burglary plot was her idea, he said. She'd seduced him into buying chloroform to knock Albert out; she'd bought the sash weight. Judd said he'd been so terrified that he'd landed only a glancing blow and then Ruth had leaped forward to finish the job. It was she who'd caught up the weight and smashed it against the side of her husband's head, dropping him to the floor. Yes, he'd helped her drag the unconscious man into bed, and yes, he'd later gone back and used the picture wire to make sure Snyder was really dead. But Gray insisted that he'd been in such a daze that he hardly remembered any of it. The fault belonged entirely to her.

At the murder trial of Ruth Snyder and Judd Gray in April, the courthouse in Queens installed fifty extra phones to accommodate the jostle of journalists. Crowds packed the streets, shoving for a glimpse of the criminals or the celebrities attending the trial. Vendors fought for the right to sell hot dogs and soda, and merchants complained that so many police officers had been diverted that neighborhood robberies had risen due to lack of patrols.

Inside the courthouse celebrities were given the coveted seats: the filmmaker D. W. Griffith, the mystery writer Mary Roberts Rinehart, the historian Will Durant, the songwriter Irving Berlin. So many Broadway entertainers attended that their benches

were dubbed "The Actors Equity Section."
Even the Marquess of Queensbury and his
wife came from England, the nobleman
claiming that he wanted to watch American
justice at first hand. At his club, the marquess said, the betting was five to one
against sexy Mrs. Snyder being convicted of
capital murder.

As a spectacle, the duo was worth it. They
spat accusations at each other. Whenever
the details became too gruesome, Ruth Snyder fainted. (She faints easily, her lawyer
explained.) Judd Gray sobbed while explaining — the police had discovered where he'd
bought the weight, the chloroform, and the
picture wire — how she'd coerced him into
doing her dirty work.

But if one looked past the lovers' theatrics
— and some, like Damon Runyon did —
the most revealing testimony came from
Alexander Gettler. In his dark suit and with
his quiet voice, he neatly dismantled both
of the accused killers' stories. He did so using only the chemistry and pathology reports that he'd brought from Bellevue.

Gettler had entered the case after the
police sent his lab the bottle of whiskey
they'd found on Judd Gray. The bottle
contained so much bichloride of mercury,
he'd discovered, that the contents were

acridly undrinkable. If Ruth Snyder had tried it on her husband, Gettler said, the man would have undoubtedly spat it out. Gettler himself had never seen such high levels of corrosive sublimate added to liquor. "Nice woman," he remarked ironically to the investigators. Gray claimed that Ruth had asked him to dispose of the bottle. But the tabloid crime reporters were enjoying theorizing that she'd been hoping her lover would take a quick nip. Newspapers began calling the trial the "Ruth versus Judd Case."

Gettler testified that Albert Snyder's brain was sodden with bootleg alcohol. The man had been woozy with drink. Gray's story — that Snyder had fought back, that Gray had been forced to defend himself with the sash weight — was simply not credible, Gettler said. The man couldn't have even been propped upright to fight. In addition, the conspirators had given Snyder a strong dose of chloroform.

The blows of the sash weight had fractured Snyder's skull, the medical examiner's office concluded, but he could have survived that. The strangling noose of the picture wire might have cut off his last breaths, but the man was already dying. Gettler's chemical analysis suggested that what really killed

Snyder was the suffocating combination of alcohol and chloroform. If his killers had left well enough alone, if they hadn't tried for the double indemnity payout, he might have appeared to die in his sleep. If they'd been just a bit smarter, just a little less greedy, they might have gotten away with it.

As it was, it took the jury only ninety minutes to find both Ruth Snyder and Judd Gray guilty of first-degree murder. On May 9, 1927, both were sentenced to die in the electric chair.

The Snyder-Gray case served as a rather pointed reminder to toxicologists such as Gettler: it was too soon to dismiss chloroform as a poisoner's tool.

A dozen years had passed since the Mors chloroform killings, but the drug continued to be used in crimes, albeit with less regularity. The previous year burglars had used chloroform to knock out a four-member Brooklyn family, emptying all valuables from the apartment as the victims lay unconscious. In September 1927 a female guest at the ornate and expensive Hotel Martinique on Broadway was drugged into unconsciousness by two robbers who then vanished with $1,600 worth of cash and jewelry.

Despite the efforts of the American Medical Association, many doctors continued to use chloroform anesthesia. It could be risky, they knew, but it was cheap and did the job. The continued demand from physicians also meant that pharmacies — as Judd Gray had found on his chloroform errand — kept it in stock.

Another reason doctors continued to use chloroform was that it remained notably difficult in the legal system to secure a conviction. In the past year two Manhattan doctors had been charged with manslaughter after their patients died under anesthesia, one an eighteen-year-old girl, the other a vaudeville actress whose husband had also brought a wrongful death suit. In both cases the physicians' colleagues successfully rallied to defend them. During the civil hearing on the actress's death, one doctor assured the jurors that he "had just been lucky" that none of his own patients had been killed by chloroform. The drug was a mystery to them all, another said. "No rules can be applied with exaction."

The physicians all decried the unpredictability of chloroform, which they pointed out usually worked well and safely. It was too bad, all agreed, that no one really knew how to measure chloroform in a body: even scientists couldn't predict when it might be lethal, couldn't measure it precisely after death to calculate a killing dose. But as it turned out, Alexander Gettler would soon get a chance to change that.

On September 15, 1927, a young woman named Ruby Gonzales came into Manhattan for a doctor's appointment. She was a waitress in Asbury Park, New Jersey, the hardworking single mother of a five-year-old girl. Gonzales brought her small daughter to the appointment as well as her boyfriend, an adding machine salesman who worked in the city.

The appointment was for an abortion, wholly illegal, wholly secret, and twenty-seven-year-old Gonzales was nervous enough to want her boyfriend for support. And really, she had no choice but to bring her daughter. All of her friends worked — they couldn't watch the child during the day. Her boyfriend had promised to get them to a hotel afterward, or somewhere she could rest and recover a little.

The two doctors running the clinic assured them all that the procedure was routine and safe. But half an hour after she arrived at the office, Ruby Gonzales was dead on the clinic table. The little girl was sobbing hysterically and the boyfriend was shouting loud enough for the neighbors to hear, such that the doctors were forced to summon the police. None of them wanted to give away that she had been there for an abortion. When the police arrived, their story was that she had started bleeding while the threesome was walking on West 10th Street, where the doctors practiced. Her boyfriend had brought her into the clinic, but she'd died before they could save her, despite all their best efforts.

Back at the morgue, the pathologists found this story, let's say, unbelievable.

They'd seen plenty of bungled abortions; this body had all the signs of a woman mangled by a hurried or incompetent doctor. She'd bled to death in the doctor's brownstone office — and no wonder. She had been shredded internally. When confronted with evidence of the abortion, both doctors shrugged the accusation away. Maybe she'd had an operation before she walked into their office, they said. She must have received the chloroform during a surgery elsewhere. They had only tried to save her. That was the substance of their statement. They saw no reason to change it.

Whether one agreed with the anti-abortion

laws or not — and in those days most did — the medical examiners were tired of doctors getting away with butchering patients. Both of these physicians had been prosecuted for botched abortions before. Judge and jury had exonerated them, apparently preferring to side with the professional man over the woman in trouble. This new death — same doctors, new victim — added to the frustration.

Gettler ran a standard toxicology analysis on the tissue from Ruby Gonzales's brain. It was loaded with chloroform; about 156 milligrams of the drug saturated every thousand grams of tissue. That was more than three times as much chloroform as had been found in the brain of Albert Snyder. Would it have killed her? It was hard to say; she'd bled to death so quickly that in one sense the anesthesia factor might be considered irrelevant.

But, while pondering the Gonzales case, Gettler realized that the chloroform results might actually be useful. They raised some interesting questions, anyway. For instance, how long did it take for chloroform to leave a brain? At what point was a patient clear-headed enough to walk down the street? If Gonzales had received the drug elsewhere, that knowledge would let them estimate how much earlier the dose had been delivered. And if the doctors had lied — as pretty much everyone in the office suspected — he might be able to prove it.

The challenge was to find those answers while the case was still active. Moving quickly, Gettler decided to run a series of animal experiments. Dogs were known to be a reliable model for studying chloroform. They responded to the drug at very similar concentrations to human beings. They also metabolized chloroform in a similar way, meaning that it cleared from their systems at about the same rate. With that knowledge, Gettler designed a straightforward test to look at response to chloroform, one that he could perform quickly enough to get some answers as to how Ruby Gonzales had died.

The department wanted the results to be inarguable, so Gettler used ten dogs, enough to check and recheck whatever he found. Each dog was tied down and a gauze mask placed over its nose and mouth. The masks were saturated with chloroform and kept in place for varying times — five minutes, half an hour, up to an hour — before being removed. The dogs were then allowed different recovery times before being killed. Some were put down while still unconscious. Others were just starting to stir, sitting up, staggering to their feet, walking in a stumble, or fully awake. At each stage the animal's brain was analyzed to see how much chloroform it retained.

One dog had died while under anesthesia, killed by the chloroform. Its brain contained 270 milligrams of chloroform per thousand grams of tissue. The still-unconscious animals had levels between 120 and 182 milligrams — directly comparable to Ruby Gonzales's brain. A dog just getting to its feet measured at 51.3 milligrams. And those that were up and walking around normally, which always took a full fifteen to thirty minutes after the chloroform mask was removed, had no more than a 30-milligram concentration of chloroform in their brains.

There was, Gettler concluded, positively no way that Ruby Gonzales could have been walking around lower Manhattan with 150-plus milligrams of chloroform in her brain. She would have been out on the table, and she would have been unconscious when she died there.

The district attorney called the two doctors back into his office and laid out the chloroform data. The doctor who ran the clinic was visibly shocked: he then admitted to the bungled abortion, and that Gonzales had been completely under when she died.

The operating physician was convicted for manslaughter and sent to Sing Sing, which, as the New York newspapers noted, didn't happen to doctors all that often.

On January 12, 1928, having lost every legal appeal, Ruth Snyder and Judd Gray went to the electric chair.

The scene around the high walls of Sing Sing prison bordered on a carnival of the macabre. Crowds of curiosity seekers arrived from as far as Chicago so as not to miss the execution of the year. Motorcars lined the street in front of the prison. Mothers stood with babies at their hips. Affectionate couples cuddled just out of the glare. Ruth Snyder's fans — she'd received 164 marriage proposals while in prison — shouted curses and pleas at the gates. Reporters jockeyed for position; one *Daily News* reporter rented an abandoned hot dog stand near the front gate and installed his own wire hookup so that he could be first to relay the news.

The prison authorities, after much vicious wrangling, provided passes for twenty journalists to view the electrocutions. Like the other witnesses, they were instructed to walk single file to the big white room that prisoners called the Death House.

In the wall opposite from where they entered was a large wooden door. The door was made of plain oak and above it hung a single sign reading: "Silence." Through that door the prisoners would enter from their quarters, an area of holding cells called the Dance House.

A few yards to the right of the oak door sat the chair itself, black metal, resting on a black metal mat. In that dark contraption a prisoner would be seated and secured in place. Straps would be buckled around the wrists, the upper arms, the chest, the waist and the ankles. Electrodes, attached to long wires and wrapped in salt water sponges to further conduct current, would be fitted to the ankles and the head. The executioner had invented the Sing Sing headgear himself: a regulation leather football helmet, lined with rubber to hold the sponge-wrapped electrodes against the head. He'd also created a mask of black leather with slits for the nose and mouth, so that no one could watch the face of a dying prisoner.

The witnesses were put in four church pews, stationed to face the chair. They sat, obeying the order for silence, waiting for the door to open.

Ruth Snyder came first, wearing a black cotton skirt and a plain brown smock. She carried a crucifix, mumbling to herself over and over, "Jesus, have mercy on me," even after the mask was put over her face. The executioner pulled the switch on the control panel, releasing a current of 2,000 volts through the wires, sending her body lurching forward against the restraints. He threw the switch twice more, just to be sure. Her hair caught fire. Her skin could be seen charring around the edges of the mask. The wardens untangled her from the chair, put her body on a gurney, and wheeled her out of the room.

Gray came next, meticulously groomed in a pinstripe suit. He waited quietly until the mask was in place and then began to recite the Twenty-third Psalm. "The Lord is my Shepherd," he murmured, "I shall not want." The executioner hit the switch. Gray's right sock began smouldering. Plumes of smoke uncoiled from under the helmet. The executioner pulled the switch again, sending another 2,000 volts. The wardens again stepped forward with their gurney. Both bodies were put into gray hearses and shuttled away for burial.

To the outrage of state officials, from the Sing Sing director to the governor, the front page of the next day's *New York Daily News* was filled by a single photo: Ruth Snyder at the moment a surge of electricity ripped through her body.

The paper had imported a famously devious photographer from Chicago's *Tribune* and sent him into the Death House posing as a writer. The photographer had a camera strapped around one leg, attached to a cable that ran up his trouser leg and into a pocket. He could squeeze a bulb in his pocket to take one picture which would be unnoticed in the glare of sparks and the horror generated by the chair.

The photographer had muscled his way into the first pew and caught an unobstructed view of Ruth Snyder's body rattling with electricity. The *Daily News* placed a single word over the photo: "Dead!" The picture was maybe a little grainy, but that only made it more exciting. The paper sold more than 1.5 million extras of that edition. Fearing that its prized photographer, Tom Howard, might be arrested, the Chicago paper sent him straight from New York to an assignment in Cuba. As he related later, a group of Marines there recognized his name — he'd become temporarily nearly as infamous as the subject of his photograph.

Howard's first thought was that the Marines had come to take him to jail. But it turned out the troops merely wanted to celebrate his Marine-worthy daring. They carted him off to a bar, where the group spent an evening cheering his success with good Havana rum. It was completely legal, after all, and the genuine article, and it tasted wonderful.

# EIGHT:
# RADIUM (Ra)
## 1928–1929

In early 1928 Norris received an unusual request for help from a fellow graduate of Columbia University's medical school, a New Jersey medical examiner named Harrison Stanford Martland.

Despite their age difference — Martland was sixteen years younger than Norris — the two men were friends as well as professional colleagues. They dined together when Martland had business in the city and sometimes went to the theater together with their wives. They bonded over a shared belief in the importance of forensics and a similar regard for their work. Like Norris, Harrison Martland was a born crusader.

Martland's medical career began in 1909, when he was named the first full-time pathologist at New York City Hospital. After the Great War started, he'd left that job to volunteer with the Bellevue Hospital unit. As a battlefield doctor, he'd proved so tireless, so determined at scraping together medical care from almost nothing, that he'd risen to the rank of lieutenant colonel and been given the job of managing a hospital in Vichy, France. When the war ended, General John Pershing himself pinned a medal on Martland, citing him for "exceptionally meritorious and conspicuous service."

After the war, Martland, the son of a Newark family practitioner, returned to his hometown and took a job as city pathologist. In 1925 he was offered the job of Essex County Physician, overseeing forensic investigations of death and illness. He accepted, only to learn that the position was in name only; the elected county coroner held all the power. If they could have worked together, Martland might have accepted that, but the coroner system turned out to be embarrassingly corrupt, much like its previous incarnation in New York City.

To the dismay of those running the political machinery in Essex County, Martland demanded real authority. In fact, he demanded that the coroner's office be replaced by a medical examiner system, along the model of Norris's office. When county executives refused, he carried his fight to the state legislature. It took two years, but in 1927 Martland was named the first chief medical examiner for Essex County.

The industrial landscape of New Jersey provided Martland with a profusion of workplace safety issues to investigate. His research helped prove that workers in explosives factories were poisoned by nitroglycerine; he wrote the first paper showing that exposure to beryllium — a flexible metallic element used in the emerging electronics industry — could lead to fatal lung diseases. Due in part to his own relentless pressure (he was a man who liked to see his research put to use), those findings would eventually result in regulatory reform.

In 1928 he was pursuing yet another industrial health hazard, one that would challenge the standard definition of a poisonous material. It was this puzzling investigation that prompted Martland to contact the New York City office. He had some aging bones in his possession, belonging to a former New Jersey factory worker. He wanted to know whether the better-equipped laboratories at Bellevue could answer this: were the bones radioactive?

To make real sense of that question, one had to look back some thirty years, to when scientists in France had announced a startling discovery. The rocks of the Earth's crust, they declared, were not all cold dead chunks of metal and mineral. Some were strangely alive. Some sizzled with energy and even emitted radiation.

The French physicist Henri Becquerel reported the first such discovery in 1896. He'd conducted experiments showing that the element uranium emitted tiny atomic particles that could pass through metal foil, creating a spatter of light spots on photographic film. Two colleagues, newly married physicists named Pierre and Marie Curie, took up Becquerel's work. Marie especially found these living rocks fascinating. Sifting through trays of ore and carefully measuring "uranium rays," she realized quickly that the emission levels were too high to be explained by the uranium alone.

After two more laborious years of sifting, testing, and recording light spatter on film, the Curies announced that they had discovered two new elements, both of which emitted particles at a greater rate than uranium. One they named polonium, after Marie Curie's native Poland. The second they simply named for radiation itself, calling it radium. They proposed that elements like radium and polonium, with their peculiar atomic snap and sizzle, should be known as "radioactive" elements.

It was radium — "my beautiful radium" as Marie called it — that seemed the most promising of these new materials. Polonium was too intensely active, burning itself away within a year. Uranium was more stable but less energized, dribbling its radiation comparatively slowly away. Radium, on the other hand, glowed with promise. It decayed slowly; its half-life was sixteen hundred years, yet it spat and sparked with a steady release of energy. The Curies had measured radium's intensity at some three thousand times that of uranium. It was rather like finding a tiny star buried in the dirt. A very tiny star — the Curies had isolated only 100 milligrams of pure radium from some three tons of uranium ore. But that gave it the allure of something truly rare.

Within two years physicians had learned that the application of radium salts to a tumor would shrink the cancer. "Radium therapy" was introduced into hospitals shortly after the turn of the twentieth century. Physicians reported healing effects that seemed miraculous, especially compared to the therapies of old. The newspapers compared radium's magic to the golden healthful rays of the sun. Everyone wanted to stand in what seemed a naturally healing light.

Radium use spread quickly into consumer products. There were bottles of radium water (guaranteed to make the drinker sparkle with energy), radium soda, radium candy, radium-laced facial creams (to rejuvenate the skin) radium-sprinkled face powder (in four clearly labeled tints: white, natural, tan, and African), soaps and pain-relieving liniments and lotions. Researchers discovered that the European hot springs, famed for their healing powers, contained radon, a gas created by an interaction of radium and water. Perhaps, scientists suggested, the health effects of the mineral hot springs came from radioactive elements in the ground. Spas in upstate New York rushed to compete by dropping uranium ores into their swimming pools. A New Jersey company grew rich selling hundreds of thousands of bottles of Radithor: Certified Radioactive Water as a tonic that guaranteed new vigor and energy.

Radiant health, the ads proclaimed — beautiful skin, endless vigor, and eternal health — ingesting radium seemed the next best thing to drinking sunlight.

Martland found radium to be neither beautiful nor inspirational.

He'd been drawn into researching it by a peculiar health crisis in Orange, New Jersey, a community just northwest of Newark. Situated on a main turnpike to Pennsylvania, Orange had long been a bustling little industrial city. It was a popular stop on the Delaware, Lackawanna, and Western railroad line. The trains made a flurry of stops at the Orange terminal, picking up and dropping off passengers, delivering Pennsylvania coal, and carrying away factory products: clocks, pencil sharpeners, boxes of shoes. Until Prohibition, the Orange Brewery had shipped its beer out on the DL&W. The old building stood dark now. But other businesses thrived in its place. The U.S. Radium Corporation, which had opened a plant there in 1917, was busier than ever.

The Radium Corporation had gotten its start in the Great War, with its new technological demands. Soldiers, huddled in the muddy trenches of Europe, learned quickly that the pocket watches they carried were unsuited to battlefields. They fell out of pockets and were crushed by the next crawling soldier; if the watches somehow weren't smashed, they were hopelessly unreadable at night. Driven by military need, watch companies began putting watches on straps, which could be safely buckled onto wrists, and they looked for a way to make watch faces glow in the dark.

Luckily, some years before the war, German scientists had developed a "self-luminous" paint. This paint glowed, due to a rather neat little cascade of chemical interactions: if radium salts were mixed with a zinc compound, particles emitted by the radium caused the zinc atoms to vibrate. The vibration created a buzz of energy, visible as a faint shiver of light. This pale greenish glow was easily outshone by daylight, but in the dark it was just luminous enough to make an instrument readable without making it easily detectable to a watching enemy.

After American troops joined the war in Europe, the factory in Orange won a contract to supply radium-dial instruments to the military. By the time the war ended, wristwatches with their glowing dials and handy wristbands were all the style. So were luminous-faced clocks, nicely dressed up in gold and ebony for elegant homes. The corporation's business was as healthy as ever — as healthy, you might say, as radium itself.

Hardly a quibble, hardly a doubt was raised, that radium might not really be the golden child of the elements.

At the factory the dial painters were taught to shape their brushes with their lips, producing the sharp tip needed to paint the tiny numbers and lines of watch dials and the lacy designs of fashionable clocks. Each worker was expected to paint 250 dials a day, five and a half days a week. They earned about twenty dollars a week for that work, at a rate of one and a half cents per completed dial.

The painters were teenage girls and young women who became friendly during their hours together and entertained themselves during breaks by playing with the paint. They sprinkled the luminous liquid in their hair to make their curls twinkle in the dark. They brightened their fingernails with it. One girl covered her teeth to give herself a Cheshire cat smile when she went home at night. None of them considered this behavior risky. Why would they, when doctors were using the same material to cure people? When wealthy spa residents were paying good money to soak in the stuff? When a neighboring company promoted the popular tonic Radithor? No one — certainly not the dial painters themselves — saw anything to worry about.

Until one by one the young workers began, mysteriously, to fall ill. Their teeth fell out, their mouths filled with sores, their jaws rotted, and they wasted away, weakened by an apparently unstoppable anemia. By 1924 nine of the dial painters were dead. They were all women in their twenties, formerly healthy, with little in common except for those hours they had spent, sitting at their iron and wood desks at the factory, painting tiny bright numbers on delicate instruments.

The bones that Martland asked Charles Norris and his staff to evaluate for radioactivity belonged to one of the first dial painters to die in Orange. Martland had ordered her body dug up and her bones sent to New York for the work. His decision got enough attention that the Newark newspaper took a picture of the New Jersey pathologist with the bones before they were sent off: a carefully posed shot of Harrison Martland with a crumbling jaw in his hand.

The industrial scandal in New Jersey foretold a change in attitude, both by scientists and by members of the public, toward radioactive elements. The change came on gradually — after all, radium had first been seen as a miracle cure. It would take more than twenty years for the element to be recognized as a killer as well as a savior.

Marie and Pierre Curie, along with Henri Becquerel, received the 1903 Nobel Prize in physics for their work with radioactive elements; Marie later donated much of her share of the prize money to the Allied war effort. She'd toured the United States, seeking money for radium research in 1921. She'd received, during that visit, the cheering welcome accorded to a woman of heroic stature.

As Curie demonstrated on her tour, she did not fear her own discovery. She kept vials of radioactive isotopes in her skirt pockets, bringing them out to show off during her lectures. She liked to see them in the dark, she'd say, to sit back and watch their pretty blue-green light. Curie was entirely reassuring about that luminous glow, but in other quarters a certain scientific wariness was surfacing regarding radium. Rumor had it that her husband, Pierre, killed in 1906 by a horse-drawn carriage, had stumbled into the street due to radiation-induced weakness. Several scientists from the European radium laboratories had developed disturbing leukemias. And when Curie finished her tour, American dignitaries presented her with a gram of radium as a gift from the United States — but it was carefully contained in a 110-pound lead box.

The occasional deaths of scientists in Europe stirred little reaction in the United States. In New Jersey, however, worries about the element grew as illness spread among the dial workers. Ironically, they began falling ill shortly after Curie's triumphant American tour. By 1924, as the painters continued to die, managers at the U.S. Radium Corporation hired a team of scientists from Harvard University to investigate the inexplicably accelerating deaths.

The Harvard scientists discovered that the watch factory was thick with radium dust. The employees were frequently covered in it. In the dark, one researcher said, the dial painters glowed like luminous ghosts. The researchers concluded that the deaths were connected to the factory work. *Connected to* rather than *caused by:* radium had a safe reputation, and they were reluctant to blame it completely. Even this cautious assessment did not go over well with factory management. The U.S. Radium Corporation refused to allow the study to be published, saying the information was too sensitive to be released.

The same year, though, a team of less co-operative scientists pursued the problem at U.S. Radium, running tests on many of the ailing workers, some still employed, others who had moved on to other jobs. The doctors from the New Jersey Consumers' League, already well known for its uncompromising positions on worker safety, published their findings, summing up with a declaration that the factory in Orange was incubating a new, strange, and terrible occupational disease.

At this point Harrison Martland decided to conduct his own investigation, one that would be uncolored by claims of pro-management or pro-worker bias. He soon agreed that radium exposure had to be the source of the problem. In his examination of the young dial painters, he'd discovered a fact that was impossible to dismiss.

The women were exhaling radon gas.

That finding provided the first real clue as to what was happening inside the workers' bodies. It also provided an early insight as to the way radium behaves, causing damage based on its naturally self-destructive nature.

The element's atomic structure is a deeply unstable one. Essentially, it exists in a state of perpetual breakdown, discarding excess parts as it decays. Subatomic particles fizz away in all directions, leaving behind an even more crazily unbalanced chemical arrangement, prone to immediate further decay. Radium is actually a breakdown product itself, created when uranium decays. Its own disintegration produces the hypercharged element polonium (sometimes called radium A) and radon gas.

Radium, then, is "radioactive" because it is constantly turning into something else, discarding unwanted parts in the form of energetic subatomic particles. The primary emissions from radium are called alpha particles; they are basically tight little bundles of protons and neutrons.

As alpha particles speed away, they take with them some of the element's energy-charged life. This high-speed flight is radiation, or alpha radiation, to be specific. Radium also emits, to a lesser degree or positrons, two other kinds of radiation: beta radiation, which consists of electrons, and gamma radiation, which contains a dangerous mixture of X-rays and other subatomic materials.

During his evaluation of the dial painter illnesses, Martland calculated that more than 90 percent of the particles shooting out of radium were alpha radiation. That wouldn't have been so bad if it had been an external exposure. Outside the body, alpha particles are rather wishy-washy bits of atomic energy. They can be stopped by a sheet of paper or a layer of clothing, even the upper layer of dead cells that overlies the skin. The two other forms of radiation are more penetrating: beta radiation easily slices through paper, although it can be stopped by a sheet of aluminum. Gamma radiation is the toughest; it takes a dense metal like lead to halt its flying particles.

But once inside the body, as Martland would soon realize, alpha radiation creates a precisely engineered internal poisoning. The radium dust noted by the Harvard team was a definite hazard because it could be inhaled. But it wasn't the source of the lethal illness among the dial painters, who were dying at a higher rate than others in the plant. The source was their practice of lip-pointing the brushes. Every time a painter put a brush in her mouth, to bring the bristles to a sharper point, she swallowed a bit of radium.

It would turn out to be the worst way to absorb the poison. Structurally, the element radium can be considered a close if crazed cousin of the element calcium. Both are alkaline earth metals, silvery white in color. Both are built in cubic crystalline structures. As a result, when a person swallows radium, the body channels it in a way similar to calcium — some is metabolized away, some goes toward nerve and muscle function, and most is deposited into the bones.

But where calcium strengthens the mineral content of the skeleton, radium does the opposite. It bombards skeletal material with alpha radiation, blasting bony material full of tiny holes, then larger ones, then larger still. It irradiates the blood-forming marrow in the bone's center. Nothing removes it until it burns itself out — and this is a material with a half-life of sixteen hundred years. Eventually Martland did find a way to get radium out of bones, but only after death: he incinerated the skeleton and then boiled the bone ashes for hours in hydrochloric acid. After that alpha radiation seemed to disappear. But otherwise, in the living body, radium spits out its alpha particles in apparently infinite supply. And its affinity for the bones explains precisely why jaws rotted away, hips broke, and ankles crumbled, why anemias and leukemias bubbled in the bone marrow.

In 1925 Martland detailed these principles of radiation poisoning in the *Journal of the*

*American Medical Association.* He'd learned many of the facts by studying the bodies of dial painters who had died. Among those still living, based on the gas they exhaled, he'd developed a formula that calculated the amount of radium in their bodies. Radon gas was produced in the skeleton as the radium there decayed; the gas diffused into the bloodstream, was carried to the lungs, and was exhaled, to drift away.

Until the next breath.

The year Martland's report was published, a small group of former employees sued U.S. Radium Corporation. Only five of the Radium Girls (as the press liked to call them) joined in that action. A few had settled, afraid to take on a big corporation, sure that they'd lose the jobs they held now, and that they'd lose in the courts as well.

These doubters knew that the company had no intention of giving in easily. It took the employees three years of legal wrangling even to get a trial date. That was why Harrison Martland called Charles Norris only in 1928 about the skeleton of a woman who had died years earlier.

The bones belonged to an Italian-American, Amelia Maggia, dead at twenty-five, who had worked as a dial painter for four years. In her last year at the factory, 1921, she'd abruptly lost weight and complained of joint pains. The following year her dentist discovered that her jaw was splintering apart; almost all of it was removed. She developed a worsening anemia and bled constantly from her mouth and died in September 1923. Her death certificate read "ulcerative stomachitis."

Martland, having found Maggia on a list of former dial painters, suspected that the diagnosis was wrong. The symptoms read like textbook radium poisoning to him. Still, the only way to prove it was to look for radiation in her skeleton, which he'd had exhumed. But he wasn't sure of the best way to test for radioactivity in these slightly decayed bones. So he wondered if the New York medical examiner's office would be willing to help him out.

Norris volunteered the time of his talented toxicologist to do the work. They were curious at Bellevue too. No one really knew that much about radium poisoning. (The title of Martland's paper was: "Some Unrecognized Dangers in the Use and Handling of Radioactive Substances.") Scientists remained unsure of what the risk was to the living and were even more uncertain about how long alpha radiation might rattle in a dead woman's bones.

The report on Amelia Maggia's bones had a title that pretty much gave away the ending: "Radioactive Substances in a Body Five Years After Death."

The paper, written by Alexander Gettler, Ralph Muller of New York University, and A. V. St. George of Bellevue's pathology laboratories, offered detailed instructions on how to take bones and tissue from an aging corpse and test them for radioactivity.

The scientists first used a knife to scrape away as many shreds of remaining tissue as possible. They burned some of those scraps into ash, then boiled a selection of bones (the skull, five cervical vertebrae, five slices of rib, both feet, both femurs, the right tibia, the right fibula) for three hours in a solution of washing soda (a slightly acidic salt known as sodium carbonate). The bones were scrubbed to dazzling white and then air-dried. The larger bones were then sawed into two-inch pieces.

Gettler and Muller next took the prepared bones into a darkroom. They had prepared their test material: X-ray films wrapped in black safety paper. The scientists placed the pieces of bone on the wrapped film and sealed everything tight to keep any stray light from interfering with the experiment. They went through the same careful procedure for the tissue ash. Then, for comparison, they went through the same process with pieces of washed bone and tissue from a normal corpse. The bone, tissue, and film packages were left to sit for ten days with the idea that "if radioactive, the bones and the tissue ash would emit rays, and the beta and gamma rays would penetrate the black paper and affect the photographic film."

After ten days they opened the packages. The published photographs showed a dazzle of pale spots, starred against a black background. "Those on which normal bones were placed are not shown, because they did not show any impression," the authors noted. As the Bellevue team reported, every bright spot was the signature of a charged particle blowing from the dial painter's bones through the protective paper onto the film. "Every piece of bone, as well as every tissue ash that we examined, showed radioactivity by the photographic method."

The report displayed Gettler's usual obsessive need to verify his results in multiple ways. He accompanied the film tests with results from experiments that relied on other techniques. He'd taken more pieces of skull, a few remnants of jaw, a vertebra, and bits of leg and foot and burned them into a gray-white ash. Scraps of tissue from the liver, lung, spleen, and brain were also weighed and incinerated.

Those ashes were placed into a radiation detector, called a Lind electroscope, and compared with comparable tissue and bone ash from another, "normal," body. The device detected alpha radiation as well as beta and gamma rays. The electroscope work confirmed the results from the film tests. Maggia's body, even after five years, was "strongly radioactive," according to the published report.

Gettler and Muller would later find an even more theatrical way to demonstrate the danger of radium in bones. In a tube attached to a Geiger counter, they placed a piece of bone from their Radium Girl. The counter *click-click-clicked* as it registered the bombardment of alpha and beta particles. The scientists connected a pair of loudspeakers to the equipment, boosting the volume of that rapid-fire rattle. In a lecture hall, the amplified crackle of radium emissions evoked the unnerving sound of enemy fire.

As the lawsuit dragged on, the five Radium Girls became sicker and sicker.

Two of them, Quinta MacDonald and Albina Larice, were sisters of Amelia Maggia, whose bones had provided so much evidence. Both of Quinta's hips had fractured. Albina was bedridden, and one of her legs was now four inches shorter than the other. Edna Hussman could barely shuffle across her room. Years after leaving the factory, her hair still glowed in the dark. Grace Fryer now worked in a bank, with a metal brace from neck to hips to support her spine. Katherine Schaub's jaws were starting to break apart; as she told her lawyers, she hoped the money — they were asking for $250,000 each — would pay for her funeral. "If I won my $250,000, mightn't I have lots of roses?"

Thirteen other dial painters, including Schaub's cousin, had died in the three years since the lawsuit was filed. But the company lawyers, in the spring of 1928, found another argument for dismissing the complaint: they proposed that the statute of limitations had run out on the plaintiffs' injuries. The workers should have come to court when they were actually exposed to radium, not now, years later, when they no longer had jobs with the U.S. Radium Corporation.

True, several of them were unemployed

because they could no longer walk or talk (as their jaws had been removed due to bone necrosis). And true, legal maneuvering had delayed proceedings. But, the company asserted, the case had lost all validity. New Jersey law required court action within two years of an injury. Some of these workers had left the factory long before the 1925 filing of the lawsuit. And so much time had passed since any workplace injury that as a matter of law, the Radium Girls' time had come and gone.

The response of the attorneys for the injured women came directly from the research publications of Harrison Martland and Alexander Gettler.

Unlike traditional toxins like arsenic or mercury, which poisoned in a single, direct dose, radium exposure inflicted a lifetime of harm. These women were still being poisoned every day by a radioactive element that never left their bodies. Yes, the suit was three years old, and yes, the women had left those dial-painting jobs years earlier. It didn't matter. All five were still exhaling radon gas and the radium in their bones was still killing them.

The judges in Newark's chancery court found the plaintiffs' argument, the image of those irreversibly radioactive bones, absolutely plausible. And appalling. The court dismissed the corporation's motion and set the trial, at last, for June 8 in federal district court in Manhattan.

Slightly more than a week later the company moved to settle the case.

The settlement was far less than the women had sought: each received only $10,000 in cash, a $400 annual pension, and the guarantee of complete medical care, to be covered by the U.S. Radium Corporation and its insurers. But they were grateful to get anything while they were still alive to use it.

The Democratic Party convention in Houston that June was, as always, an excellent party. All enjoyed it except for the New York delegates, who had very specific instructions to behave and not to drink in public. As humorist Will Rogers, who was covering the conference, wrote, the New Yorkers were pitiful, just pitiful. "They all say 'Why pick on us to be the only sober ones here?' "

The answer to that was obvious. New York governor Al Smith had a real chance at the presidential nomination. He also had two major political liabilities. He was a Catholic in a country dominated by Protestants, which couldn't be changed. And he had a reputation as an enemy of Prohibition, even as a man in the pocket of the bootleggers. That could at least be minimized.

In Rogers's words, "The whole talk down here is wet and dry; the delegates just can't wait till the next bottle is opened to discuss it." Smith suspected that being seen as a drinker's friend was no longer as much of a handicap as it had been a few years earlier; the Democrats might even position themselves as the party opposed to punitive alcohol regulations.

By the convention's end, aided by his alcohol-deprived colleagues, Smith had succeeded in his quest and was the Democratic candidate for U.S. President. In the November election he would face Commerce Secretary Herbert Hoover, a reform-minded Republican backed by pro-Prohibition partisans.

As the election approached, Rogers's perspective on the nation's illicit love affair with alcohol lost some of its lightheartedness. In a letter to the *New York Times*, musing on the perpetual danger now posed by drinking with friends, he wrote: "This 'speakeasy' business must be the most independent and prosperous business in the world, especially in New York, for no other industry in the world could afford to kill its customers off like that. They must run an undertaking business on the side."

The first October weekend, four New Yorkers were killed and eleven were sickened by poisoned alcohol; the following weekend another eleven were dead and sixty hospitalized. Norris issued yet another warning: "Practically all the liquor that is sold in New York today is toxic," because practically all the liquor was redistilled denatured alcohol. "Whether they call it smoke, or white mule or put in some flavoring and call it gin, the effect is the same."

Two days later another twenty-two people were dead.

Mayor Jimmy Walker was famously fond of the speakeasy lifestyle, earning himself the nickname "Night Mayor." But even he had had enough. On October 8 he angrily demanded a sweep of backroom bars on the Lower East Side, the source of the recent cascade of deaths, and that an example be made: "I do insist that those responsible for this poison liquor, the sale of which amounts to a homicide and which is more than a violation of the Volstead act, be apprehended and prosecuted."

For his part, Norris put most of the blame elsewhere. Gettler's latest tests had found the lethal bite not only of methyl alcohol but of the government's determined, ever-expanding use of poisonous additives: aldehol, pyridine, benzene, diethyl phlatate, nicotine, mercury, aniline, phenols.

"Prohibition is a joke," Norris said flatly. "I invite both Presidential candidates to see the noble experiment in extermination. The medical examiners cannot stop these deaths. It is up to the authorities to stop them."

In November 1928, Herbert Hoover won forty of the forty-eight states, including New York. Smith took Massachusetts and Rhode Island, both with large Catholic populations, and a small cluster along the Gulf Coast. The southern states had been swayed to Smith by deliberately spread, and untrue, rumors that Hoover favored integration of schools. But rumors manufactured by his opponent had taken a greater toll on Smith. Throughout the election he was forced to counter claims that he took his orders first from the Vatican, then from Tammany Hall, and then from gangsters who wanted to preserve their bootlegging profits.

Although the governor failed to carry his home state, he did win in New York City, where crooked politics were nothing new, and where an anti-Prohibition stand was considered next to godliness.

In October 1929, Marie Curie made another radium tour of the United States. Again she was welcomed as the most famous woman scientist of her time.

In the eight years since her first visit, radium had lost some of its popular luster. The Public Health Service was investigating the health hazards of radium dial painting, looking beyond New Jersey to watch making factories in Ohio and Connecticut. Curie herself was less ebullient about her favorite element, cautioning that radium could after all be dangerous and recommending that only experts handle it.

She suffered from an unusual state of dragging exhaustion on this trip, expressing gratitude to the press for its "generosity in excusing me from interviews and photographs because of my physical condition." Still, even if the intervening decade had raised doubts about the element radium, its discoverer was considered a woman to celebrate. She was a pioneer, the rare woman of the early twentieth century to triumph in science, a researcher whose discovery had transformed both physics and chemistry.

During her second radium tour, Curie

went to a dinner for Thomas Edison, hosted by Henry Ford; she planted a "radium maple" in a park in Westchester County; the New York City Women's Federation awarded her their medal of honor; and she dedicated the Hall of Chemistry at St. Lawrence University, where she received an honorary degree. Naturally, she took the train down to Washington, D.C., to be feted at the White House, where President Hoover praised her "beneficent service to mankind."

At the end of her month-long visit, she sailed back home on the *Ile de France,* bearing another gram of radium, worth $50,000, given to her by her American admirers and once again packed deep inside a box of lead. But the exhaustion that had plagued her did not relent. And eventually, Marie Curie fell victim to her beautiful radium. She died in 1934 of aplastic anemia, a disease caused when bone marrow is so damaged that it can no longer renew the body's supply of blood cells. It was the same anemia that had killed so many of the Radium Girls.

Curie's second radium fling in the United States ended just before the country slid into an economic crisis. Barely a week after she sailed for France, the New York Stock Market crashed. Stock prices fell for days, bottoming out on October 29, which would be forever after remembered as "Black Tuesday." Financial losses totaled some $30 billion in less than a week, more than the country had spent in all of the Great War.

The business scandals, the threat of bank failures, and the flurry of suicides followed almost immediately. At the medical examiner's office they could literally count the collateral damage — the head of a produce firm who jumped out a seventh-floor window on Wall Street, the broker who swallowed poison in his home, the banker who threw himself under a truck, the bookkeeper who drowned himself. In the midst of that eddying cycle of panic and death, Norris made what he always considered one of his worst mistakes as medical examiner.

Late on the night of Friday, November 9, J. J. Riordan, head of the County Trust Company, shot himself in the head. Norris was notified early Saturday morning, not long after Riordan's widow had found the body and started making phone calls. These were highly placed phone calls. It was a friend of former governor Al Smith who contacted the medical examiner. Smith had left public office after losing the national election and was now president of a corporation which was preparing to build a monumental skyscraper, to be called the Empire State Building. But the former governor still had strong allies in city government. His associate arrived at Norris's Upper West Side home driving a fire truck to convey the medical examiner to the banker's home. Smith himself met Norris at the door and took him to the banker's study.

Riordan's body was still sitting in a red-plush chair. The crimson fabric helped disguise the blood that had saturated the chair, but the right side of the man's once-white shirt was now a browning scarlet. The dead banker's forehead was smudged black around a hole just over the right eyebrow. Norris leaned over and felt for an exit wound; there was none. Pressing harder around the skull, he could feel the bullet lodged against cracked bone on the left side of the head; it had plowed through the brain before stopping just inside the skull.

Where was the gun? he asked. Riordan's wife admitted to prying it away from her husband's hand and hiding it. Norris demanded its return. The gun was a five-chambered Colt .38 revolver, with all chambers loaded but one. He bagged the weapon, finished his notes, and prepared to return to the office to write his report. As he recalled later, it was at that moment that

Norris belatedly realized why Al Smith was there, and why he himself had been conveyed in such secrecy.

The "ex-Governor was the principal spokesman" in a plea to hold back the announcement of the death. Specifically, the officials gathered around Norris wanted a delay until the close of banking hours on Saturday at noon. They needed the time, he was told, to make sure the accounts were in order. Everyone feared a bank run; news of bank closures seemed to arrive daily from elsewhere in the country, from Chicago, from Miami, from Los Angeles. The following year the banking crisis would arrive in New York City, shutting down hundreds of savings institutions; already the shrill of panic was sounding in the air.

So Norris agreed to hold off on his findings. After Riordan's bank closed for the day, he went to personally inform the police commissioner and to turn over the telltale revolver. But despite all precautions, the little conspiracy leaked to the newspapers, embarrassing them all. No one apparently more than Norris — he was, at least, the only member of the cover-up to apologize publicly.

It had been a mistake, he later said. He'd been persuaded that he needed to help avoid a banking panic but he should have shown more respect for the good citizens who patronized the Country Trust Company. The result of the Riordan fiasco, he feared, was more mistrust, a sense that the medical examiner's office was willing to conspire with the city's elite. "I accept responsibility for the delay," Norris said in a spare public statement that helped put an end to the controversy.

But the chief medical examiner remained furious with all concerned, especially himself for going along with the scheme: "The chief kept his peace publicly, but he had quite a lot to say privately, and his language was picturesque and to the point," city pathologist Edward Marten later recalled. Norris blamed himself for forgetting one of his cardinal rules, that medical examiners should never be swayed by politicians. He wouldn't forget again.

# NINE:
## ETHYL ALCOHOL
## $(C_2H_5OH)$
### 1930–1932

From the records of Alexander O. Gettler:

CASE 1: A moderate drinker, aged 25, in apparent good health, wagered that he could drink 1 pint of whiskey within ten minutes. He drank one-and-a-half pints of cheap whiskey and started for home. He soon became unconscious, vomited, and became comatose. His face was livid, he breathed heavily, and after four or five convulsions, he died six hours from time of drinking the spirits. At autopsy, undigested liquor still in stomach, pupils widely dilated and unequal, brain saturated with blood, lungs spotted with hemorrhages.

CASE 2: Woman, aged 41, a periodic inebriate, drank one and a half pints of exceptionally strong whiskey. Found lying on back insensible in a few minutes, died five and a quarter hours later without recovering consciousness. On autopsy: pupils were dilated, patches of mucous membrane of the stomach were found semi-detached; parts of stomach walls were fiery red.

CASE 3: Laborer aged 33, drank between 10 and 15 ounces of whiskey. He became intoxicated in 20 minutes, and fell to the ground in a deep sleep soon afterward. It was impossible to rouse him. The pupils were contracted to almost pinpoint size; death took place nineteen hours later. Autopsy, thirty hours after death: body completely stiff with rigor mortis, brain congested with blood.

All three deaths wove together in a pattern recognizable to any forensic chemist. The party boy, the old alcoholic, and the drunken laborer — none of them, as Gettler's analyses would prove, died from imbibing the notoriously dangerous methyl alcohol. They'd been killed instead by so-called good liquor: whiskey made intoxicating and toxic by ethyl alcohol.

Thanks to the government's deliberate poisoning of alcoholic spirits people had seemingly forgotten that liquor had always been dangerous. There was a reason that beverages containing ethyl alcohol were known as "hard liquor," that its consumption, or overconsumption, had driven the outrage that led to Prohibition, that its history was threaded with destructive behavior from addiction to street brawls, and that it had killed many more people than methyl alcohol ever would.

"From almost every standpoint ethyl alcohol must be regarded as the most important poison with which medical men and jurists have to deal," Gettler wrote in a paper, listing a seemingly endless record of fatalities. "No other poison causes so many deaths or leads to or intensifies so many diseases, both physical and mental, as does [this] alcohol in the many forms in which it is taken."

Ever the research chemist, Gettler believed it was time, past time, to start understanding exactly how ethyl alcohol compromises a human body. He especially wanted to study its effects on the brain. "In a nation trying to enforce alcoholic prohibition, it would seem unwarranted to do any research work on the alcoholic content of human organs," he added. But he would do it anyway. The dry crusaders in the federal government might believe this work was unnecessary, but the new generation of forensic toxicologists knew better.

So did the country's insurance agencies. Their findings came from statistics rather than test tubes, but the conclusions were remarkably similar.

In early 1930 the Metropolitan Life Insurance Company reported that deaths due to alcoholism were now 600 percent higher (among its 19 million policyholders) than those tallied in 1920, the first year that consumption of alcohol was prohibited. These statistics suggested that Prohibition had fostered a nation of heavy drinkers and that the habit was killing thousands of people.

Prudential Life Insurance reported the same disheartening trend: at the start of Prohibition, the company's records showed a national rate of about 1,000 deaths a year due to acute alcoholism. That number now approached 5,000. These numbers reflected only the company's policyholders, but Prudential's chief statistician had extrapolated to estimate that about 3 in every 100,000 Americans now died from acute alcoholism. In the wettest state in the country, New York, the death rate was 7.5

per 100,000. In only one other place were people drinking themselves to death at a comparable rate: Washington, D.C., where the laws creating this particular chapter in the history of Gettler's "most important poison" had been written.

Alexander Gettler had another reason, though, for exploring the chemistry of ethyl alcohol. It was an important poison, absolutely, but it was also a fascinating one. It offered an illuminating case study in the peculiar, paradoxical nature of the planet's chemistry: what sustained life could also kill it.

Arguably the three most important atoms on Earth are carbon, oxygen, and hydrogen. Carbon provides the fundamental chemical base of every life-form on the planet, past and present. When fuels derived from the decomposed and fossilized life of the past — such as coal or gasoline — burn, they release carbon into the air. Oxygen is vital to keeping carbon-based life forms alive, barring a few odd creatures like anaerobic bacteria. And if two hydrogen atoms attach to a single oxygen atom, the result — $H_2O$ — is that gloriously necessary liquid called water.

Mixed together, rearranged, and stretched

out into long chains, elaborate arrangements, and simple atomic blocks, these three chemicals write the story of life on Earth. They form sugars, proteins, acids, hormones, enzymes — the list is nearly endless. That complex list also includes the familiar and risky family of alcohols.

The primary alcohols, including methyl and ethyl, are straightforward arrangements of carbon, hydrogen, and oxygen. In the curious way of chemistry, the deadlier of the two compounds is more simply constructed. Methyl alcohol is $CH_3OH$. It begins with a cluster of three hydrogen atoms encircling one of carbon. That cluster is firmly linked to an oxygen-hydrogen pair called a hydroxyl radical. Ethyl is a slightly bulkier compound: $C_2H_5OH$. Two carbons and five hydrogens form a chunky arrangement, once again attached to that highly reactive hydroxyl radical.

Some fancier alcohols have more complicated structures, containing, for instance, more carbon atoms. But such elaborate alcohols were never destined to become the stuff of drinking legends, the magic ingredient in a golden brandy and soda, a copper-hued scotch and water, because they aren't water soluble. It turns out that the extra carbon interferes with the molecular mixing process. (Others, like isopropyl alcohol, also known as rubbing alcohol, dissolve into salt-free water but separate when mixed into a saline solution.)

The wonderfully soluble, amazingly intoxicating ethyl alcohol, derived from the fermentation of fruits, grains, and even vegetables, is by far the most popular member of the alcohol family. And the most thoroughly studied. Research interest in ethyl alcohol dates back to the eighth century, when alchemists working for the caliph of Baghdad started experimenting with distillation methods, leaving behind detailed observations on the flammable vapors of boiled wine.

A good thousand years later scientists in nineteenth-century England identified ethyl alcohol's chemical formula, learned to synthesize it and make it on an industrial scale. Mass-produced ethyl alcohol (also called ethanol) has uses far beyond potable spirits. Denatured, it can be used for everything from solvents to fuel. Even automobiles can run on alcohol; in fact, until Prohibition, the Model T Ford could be, and often was, adapted to run on ethanol. The practice fell out of favor once bootleggers started siphoning off the fuel from cars and repackaging it and the government enforcement division charged ethanol manufacturers with enabling criminal activities.

Before Prohibition most people wouldn't have considered drinking fuel alcohol. They had a choice of good corn whiskies like bourbon, grain alcohols from beer to scotch, hard apple cider, and fermented grape products from wine to brandy. When those drinks were legal, the government regulated the amount of alcohol they could contain. Beer, for instance, usually contained 2 to 6 percent alcohol, wine from 7 to 20 percent, and whiskey 40 percent. Bootlegged whiskey was a different matter. Some of the bottles confiscated by the police and analyzed at the Bellevue laboratories were 60 percent alcohol (a staggering 120 proof). And some were nothing but alcohol.

Depending on one's perspective, it was one of the benefits, or curses, of ten years of Prohibition: every drink was a stiff one.

That description took on an ironic meaning when considering corpses of those killed by ethyl alcohol. The cadavers tended, for reasons not quite clear to the pathologists, to stiffen in death, sometimes remaining rigid for days, while the other bodies in the morgue softened like wax on a summer day.

Perhaps, the medical examiners speculated, that was because the high alcohol content suffusing the bodies preserved them, even pickled them. As Gettler once noted, it takes a determined drinker to imbibe a lethal amount of ethyl alcohol. The liquid lacks the viciously subversive makeup of its chemical cousin, methyl alcohol. If the two were a little more alike, frankly, alcohol consumption would never have caught on.

When the enzymes in the liver break apart methyl alcohol, the result is the two poisons formic acid and formaldehyde. Ethyl alcohol, by contrast, dissolves rather easily into acetic acid, the bitter but basically harmless compound that is the primary constituent in vinegar, and the acid breaks down further into carbon dioxide and water.

The graceful disintegration of ethyl alcohol means that, in moderate amounts, it usually metabolizes out of the body without causing any immediate harm or even calling much attention to itself. The risk increases, of course, with continual exposure. Like most alcohols, ethyl is an irritant — too much will inflame the stomach enough to induce nausea and vomiting. It also causes dehydration: "alcohol abstracts water from the tissues and precipitates proteins," in

Gettler's careful phraseology. Chronic drinking, chronic irritation and dehydration can eventually lead to long-term damage, especially to the liver, which does most of the work in breaking down the alcohol so that it can be moved out of the body.

As the pathologists in Charles Norris's department discovered, people who chugged ethyl alcohol often didn't live long enough to develop the signs of chronic liver destruction. Their autopsies revealed different damage: the stomach and esophagus were a deep, irritated red; tiny blooms of blood patterned the mucous lining of the stomach; the brain was bruised-looking and flushed with excess blood.

The last fact caught Gettler's attention, reminding him that alcohol crosses the blood-brain barrier. But what does it actually *do* once it permeates the brain? For all the bodies gathered up over the years, for all the drinkers scraped off city sidewalks, no one really knew the answer to that question.

For Gettler and the young chemists studying with him — a next generation of toxicologists who would become known in the profession as the Gettler Boys — the alcohol-poisoned cadavers, those literal stiffs, raised question after intriguing question.

Pathologists routinely found the bloody evidence of ethyl alcohol damage in bodies collapsed on sidewalks or in stairwells. The city toxicologists routinely extracted alcohol from blood and brain. But they had no way to attach meaning to it. No one had figured out how much alcohol in the blood meant intoxication, much less how to calculate what various alcohol levels in the brain meant. The basic assumption was that of common sense: the higher the alcohol level in the blood, the greater the probable state of drunkenness.

On the other hand, sometimes one person would appear to be intoxicated by a small amount of alcohol while another would seem remarkably steady even after enjoying a bounty of whiskey or a buffet of cocktails. People might talk of hard heads and experienced drinkers, but such variances made it very difficult for pathologists to figure out whether a man or woman was genuinely impaired by alcohol at the time of death.

Gettler reasoned that the presence of alcohol in the blood wasn't true evidence of drunkenness: the bloodstream didn't affect behavior. It delivered materials to organs, like the brain, that did so. Equally logically, liquor found still sloshing in the stomach could have no impact at all. "It indicates merely that alcohol has been partaken of, but can in no way be taken as an index of intoxication," Gettler wrote.

The answer had to lie in the correlation between alcohol levels in the blood and in the brain: how much meant cheerful intoxication, and how much meant falling-down drunk? Along with his Gettler Boys, he decided that now was the right moment to solve the problem, and the fact that they were studying an illegal substance, in the midst of Prohibition, didn't bother them at all.

The blues songs telling of poison started in 1930. From Tennessee came a mournful plaint of paralysis, a man who couldn't walk or talk after drinking with friends. From Wisconsin sounded a bitter ode to the drink Ginger Jake. The writer worried that everyone he knew was now messed up by the cocktail.

The same year, from Mississippi, singer Willie "Poor Man" Loftus wailed, "Mama cried out and said, Oh Lord, there's nothin' in the world poor daddy can do, 'cause he done drank so much jake, he done got the limber leg, too."

From Brooklyn arose another kind of sound — the angry crash of a raid, that May of 1930, when enraged Prohibition agents arrested a local operator who'd concocted a uniquely poisonous alcoholic drink in his small factory — barrels and barrels of Ginger Jake, shipped to southern states, the very drink that had inspired all those mournful songs.

Mr. Walter Anderson, of Brooklyn's Decker, Ingraham & Smith Pharmaceuticals, wasn't the only operator making Ginger Jake or even the biggest swindler. Some of the larger Jake rings, investigators would discover, operated out of St. Louis and Cincinnati. But Anderson, by selling his mixture wholesale at $225 a barrel, putting it into two-ounce bottles that sold for thirty-five cents in drugstores, candy stores, and roadside stands, purveyed along with the ice cream and the pre-cut sandwiches, was getting rich enough.

Jake was based on an old patent medicine, Jamaican Ginger, which was really ginger-flavored ethyl alcohol, between 70 and 80 percent by weight. Following the passage of the Eighteenth Amendment, the government had ordered Jamaican Ginger makers, like Anderson's Brooklyn company, to reduce the alcohol and double the ginger.

This Prohibition-approved recipe turned out to be a money-losing proposition, turning the concoction from a popular tonic (especially among those looking for a cheap drink) to a horribly bitter black syrup.

Anderson's license to make Jamaican Ginger had been revoked a year earlier, when Treasury tests showed he was spiking his product with extra alcohol. It became obvious that he hadn't shut down, merely started another operation in secret, pretending to be making aftershave lotions while cooking up his lucrative supplies of Ginger Jake.

Bootleggers had fiddled with Jamaican Ginger substitutes over the years, trying to keep them as cheap as possible. The new Jakes usually contained bottom-of-the-barrel ingredients — one short-lived formula included creosote and carbolic acid. But in early 1930, a pair of syndicate chemists from Boston found a better recipe, one based on an industrial compound known as a plasticizer, which was easy enough to steal from George Eastman's Kodak Company in Rochester, New York, or from the Celluloid Company of Newark, New Jersey. It was this improved version that Anderson, among others, had adopted.

The new additive was a compound used

to keep plastics, such as those in photographic film, from becoming brittle. It combined those standard atoms — carbon, hydrogen, and oxygen — with phosphorus; its technical name was tri-o-cresyl phosphate. The name explains the structure: carbon, hydrogen, and oxygen bond into a ring-shaped structure called a cresol (also found in creosote), and phosphorus hangs on to the ring like an exhausted swimmer gripping a life preserver.

In the new Jamaican Gingers the plasticizer combined with denatured alcohol to form a compound called an organophosphate. That potent combination was responsible for Jake's newly powerful buzz. The dizzying sensation derived from the fact that the compound was also an efficient neurotoxin — as became almost immediately and horrifyingly evident.

The Jake Leg epidemic, as people would call it, began in February 1930 with a sudden, inexplicable spate of paralysis cases in Oklahoma City. Doctors there first feared they were witnessing an outbreak of polio. But the men suddenly crowding into city hospitals, sixty-five in a single week, showed none of the predictable symptoms of that dread infection — the fever and stiffness, the muscle spasms and difficulty swallowing and breathing. They simply and in the strangest way began to lose control of their hands and feet.

Some victims of this peculiar new outbreak could walk all right, but they had no control over the muscles that normally positioned the feet. They developed what came to be called the "jake walk": raising their feet high, the toes flopping downward. Point toes, step, heel down, point toes — the men made a distinctive *tap-click, tap-click* sound as they walked. Other muscles flopped as well — the muscles below the knee, the ones that connected fingers and thumbs. But it was the tapping walk that gave the syndrome its best-known and most bitter nicknames: jake leg, jake foot, jakeitis, jakeralysis, and gingerfoot.

By summer, physicians across the country were reporting the results of the handiwork of Jake dealers like the Brooklyn company: thousands of paralysis cases fanned across the South and Southwest, where Jamaican Ginger had made up a cheap cocktail, mixed with ginger ale, for many years. The Public Health Service counted more than two thousand Jake cases in Mississippi alone, nearly as many in Kansas, hundreds more in Kentucky, Oklahoma, Tennessee, Georgia, and Texas, and even an odd few in

Rhode Island and Massachusetts.

It took months for scientists to identify the plasticizer; they first suspected creosote, then carbolic acid, before they untangled the Ginger Jake chemistry. And when they realized that the crippling agent was the plasticizer, they were genuinely surprised. Organophosphates weren't considered all that dangerous. Now Ginger Jake forced public health chemists to somewhat reluctantly reassess that idea. The studies that followed the epidemic, both through autopsies and through animal studies (in Oklahoma, the scientists did the work in chickens), showed that the compound was horrifyingly precise in its action. It chewed through a specific series of nerve cells in the spinal cord, the anterior horn cells. These were motor neurons; researchers would later find that people suffering from ALS suffered damage in these same cells.

But Ginger Jake hardly dampened enthusiasm for a very promising new group of industrial chemical compounds that people usually didn't drink. It would be decades before another organophosphate, the broad-spectrum pesticide DDT, startled the public into realizing how risky such chemistry could be. The pesticide became the subject of a scientific manifesto, Rachel Carson's

*Silent Spring,* and helped trigger an environmental revolution in the United States.

In New York City, where the preferred drink of 1930 was bootleg gin, the Jake epidemic proved mostly a curiosity, barring some unwanted attention paid to Brooklyn's innovative chemical manufacturers.

After busting Anderson and his Ginger Jake factory, dry agents discovered a liquor distribution ring that was cleverly using the cosmetics industry as a cover. For this project the chemist had purchased perfumes from around the country, stripped them down to the raw alcohol, boosted their intoxication factor with the same plasticizer used in Ginger Jake, repackaged the alcohol as perfume, and sent the packages to druggists, who sold them from under the counter to customers in the know, who unfortunately also developed a sinking paralysis.

The head of the syndicate — identified by the government as Harry Mandell, alias Charles Harris, alias Ralph Lewis of Brooklyn — had put together an enviable national network. By the time the government finished hunting down his co-conspirators, more than one hundred druggists had been indicated in Kansas alone, along with Harris-Lewis-Mandell and seventeen other

Brooklyn residents.

James Doran, director of the Treasury Department's Bureau of Industrial Alcohol, used the moment to remind the American drinking public that bootleggers were not their friends. Members of the alcohol syndicates, he suggested, would poison their mothers to make money. They were criminals, liars, and businessmen "evidently operating on a get-rich-quick basis."

That "get rich" part was all bootleggers cared about and all they ever would. And on that point, even Charles Norris and Alexander Gettler agreed with him — a rare moment of consensus between the medical examiner's office and the Prohibitionist Doran.

By 1930, Gettler had assembled an encyclopedic list of cases for his research into the chemistry of drunkenness. Back in the 1920s he and one of his trainees, a promising chemist named Arthur Tiber, had begun that project on an optimistic note — they had an unlimited supply of test subjects since "intoxicated people were encountered every day" on the streets and alcoholic deaths were logged into the morgue every night.

Once again Gettler was in the right department, the right building, and just the right job for this kind of research. The morgue was a repository of alcohol victims, accident victims, people shot to death, people drowned, and those claimed by illness and age. He had bodies to test for alcohol levels, and he had bodies to use for comparison purposes. When he tallied up his project, he found it had consumed more than five years of research and some six thousand brains.

The work could best be described as gruesomely tedious.

To establish baseline numbers, Gettler and Tiber would mince chunks of brain from people who had died of natural causes, sometimes using as much as half a pound of gray matter per test. They'd distill the gory sludge of tissue with steam, eventually collecting a clearish pink fluid. That fluid would be divided in half; they'd set one sample aside and test the other. Then they'd divide the remaining half into halves and test one portion of that. Again and again they would test and then retest these divisions, which chemists liked to call aliquot portions, dividing and redividing, trying to figure out how small a sample would still tell them what they wanted to know.

Gettler's steam distillation apparatus used

a two-liter flask, where steam was generated, connected by glass tubes to a second vessel that contained the brain tissue. From there more glass tubes led to a condensing unit and then to a glass container that collected the dripping fluid of the final product. The whole assemblage was almost eight feet long and was housed under a hood. Eventually, as need for the tests grew, Gettler would fill an entire room of his laboratory quarters with the oversize alcohol-analysis devices.

Each apparatus worked by mimicking the way the human body metabolizes ethyl alcohol into acetic acid. If a tissue sample contained alcohol, the acid would form in that spiderweb of glass tubes and drip into the last collection flask. If Gettler was working with a large quantity of alcohol, he didn't need such elaborate measures; he could find ethyl alcohol more directly. But he was hunting for a way to find traces of the compound at a level long thought undetectable. Analyzing bare smears of brain tissue, he'd learned that the acetic acid test offered the most sensitive measurement available.

In the third-floor laboratory Gettler and his assistants duplicated the tests until they were sure of one fact: the tissue of a normal brain always contains a trace of ethyl alcohol as a result of normal metabolic processes. And *trace* was the right word: at most, natural alcohol content in the brain is 2/1,000th of a percent.

But that number, that barest gleam of alcohol, gave them a baseline reading to compare to the brains of people who had consumed alcohol. That was the real question anyway — how much alcohol was added when people drank, when they drank a little, and when they drank way too much? How much did it take before the brain was, one might fairly say, soaking in the stuff?

"Well, Doctor, isn't it a fact that I can give the same amount of alcohol to two people, and one may become intoxicated and the other not?" Gettler was forever being asked that question by attorneys representing clients charged with public intoxication or drunk driving or any of the alcohol offenses that had continued, without fail, to plague the criminal justice system during Prohibition.

"My answer to that is, we are not analyzing what the man gets to drink." As he'd said for years, he didn't care about that, didn't care what was in the bottle, the stomach, or the intestines, didn't even fully count the blood-alcohol level. "We are analyzing for the alcoholic content of the brain. Once it gets to the brain, it has an effect, and that effect is proportionate to the amount present" in those tissues.

To correlate the amount of alcohol in the brain with drunken behavior, Gettler had pored over the remains of people identified as drunk at time of death, people who'd fractured their skulls falling down stairs, meandered in front of a hurrying automobile or tumbled onto train tracks and been collected in pieces. He'd matched them to witness statements gathered by the police, descriptions of those weaving, stumbling, and joking their way toward their final conclusion. For comparison, he'd also looked at the brains of people who'd consumed no alcohol, patients who'd died at Bellevue after lengthy hospitalizations, people whose tissues were guaranteed to contain no more than the normal baseline of ethyl alcohol.

All of that — the measurements of alcohol in the brain, the injuries, the behavior, the full context of those deaths — would go into the paper that he and Tiber published, which would be widely acclaimed as creating the first scientific scale of intoxication.

Gettler's scale used the numerical plus

sign + to indicate each level of drunken-ness. Each plus stood for a level above normal: baseline brain alcohol plus one, plus two, plus three, or plus four. Spelled out, the scale read like this:

+ "In all cases in which there was an alcoholic content of the brain below 0.1 percent, the patients showed no obvious alcohol impairment."

++ From 0.1 to 0.25 percent alcoholic content. Subjects showed slight inebria-tion: they were a little more aggressive than normal, a little less cautious in their behaviors. One man who had knocked back a couple of drinks, pitched into a bar fight, and was stabbed to death had a ++ rating.

+++ From 0.25 to 0.4 percent alco-holic content. In the hours before death, subjects were unsteady on their feet, loud, and judged drunk by everyone who saw them. A typical +++ was autopsied after he'd fallen down the stairs while drunk and broken his neck.

++++ From 0.4 to 0.6 percent alco-holic content. These subjects had died after becoming falling-down drunk. They had consumed so much liquor that they succumbed to ethyl alcohol poisoning, usually within several hours after reaching a hospital.

Gettler's one-to-four scale of drunkenness was ideal for establishing intoxication at time of death, working as it did with brain tissue.

A companion rating scale — for the drunk drivers who survived a crash — would follow shortly. In 1931, an Indiana University toxicologist named Rolla Harger invented the "Drunk-o-Meter," a device in which drinkers blew into a balloon, allowing chemists to analyze the vapors in their breath. Harger's system, like Gettler's, assigned intoxication values linked to behaviors measured at each level of chemical results.

The Prohibition era had been a great source of material for building an excellent science of alcohol intoxication.

In New York City, according to press reports, two men in a First Avenue speakeasy died from alcohol poisoning in August. Six died and twenty-one were hospitalized in September, all sickened by wood alcohol served in a Brooklyn bar. In October another twenty were dead in Newark. They'd apparently skipped the redistilling process entirely and guzzled straight industrial alcohol.

In December 1930 James Doran acknowledged that the death rate was worsening, at least for "a certain type of person with uncontrollable appetite." The latest holiday drink was a mixture that included the alcohol used in antifreeze formulas. The antifreeze cocktail was a favorite of rail riders, traveling laborers who liked to sneak their rides on cargo trains. They called the drink "derail" for its near-instant brand of intoxication. It killed a few of them, sure, but they were used to the effects of borderline alcohol. The rail riders admitted — or sometimes boasted — that they'd drunk Sterno on occasion, or bay rum aftershave if there was nothing else to be found.

"These deaths have been attributed to so-called poison liquor," Doran acknowledged, "namely denatured alcohol, manufactured under government supervision." In response to continued criticism — Charles Norris had taken to describing the United States as the land of hypocrisy — Prohibition chemists had invented a new formula, to be introduced in 1931, which they thought would be repulsive without actually killing people.

The new formula mixed petroleum products into the alcohol, pretty much the sludge left behind during gasoline processing. Noxious with the rotten-egg reek of hydrogen sulfide, they figured it would be unpleasant enough to discourage anyone conscious enough to get a whiff. To publicize the new approach, the Treasury Department invited journalists to come taste it. One experienced newshound immediately identified it as containing either benzene or ether. "It's not as bad as some of the stuff you've been drinking," Doran replied ironically, as the writer, clearly accustomed to the more usual versions of poisoned alcohol, chugged down another sample.

Why were some people, journalists notoriously among them, seemingly able to guzzle alcohol without obvious effect? Why didn't everyone fall flat after a marathon of martinis? These questions were asked enviously by hungover friends, resentfully by dry advocates. And they had perplexed scientists for decades.

Gettler could — and did — cite puzzled research papers dating back to the turn of the century. One of the most provocative, published in 1908, was a study of rats and rabbits that were provided a regular supply of ethyl alcohol. After the scientists had created a colony of alcoholic animals, they offered the same laboratory cocktails to animals with no previous exposure. The novice drinkers became stumbling drunk on the same amount of alcohol that no longer had any effect on the habituated rats and rabbits.

By doing a series of blood draws, the scientists found that their habitués had somehow learned to better process their drinking binges. The unaccustomed animals absorbed 20 percent more alcohol into their bloodstream in the first two hours than did the practiced ones. By the end of a day, first-time drinkers had blood-alcohol levels 66 percent higher than the experienced imbibers.

Working with his talented toxicology students, Abe Freireich (who would later become chief medical examiner for New York's Nassau County), Gettler decided to see if he could provide a better understanding of how alcohol is metabolized by different kinds of drinkers. He chose dogs for their experiments.

Gettler and Freireich assembled a research colony of twenty-four animals, half destined to become canine alcoholics. They started by giving those twelve dogs drinks that were

98 percent water and 2 percent ethyl alcohol. Over the next two months the alcohol portion was increased to 30 percent. When Gettler and Freireich were sure that their dogs were habituated to alcohol, they started the actual experiment; it would continue for two years before they were satisfied with the results.

They started simply, comparing the effects of alcohol on a dog accustomed to ethyl alcohol to one that had never touched it before. Both animals were given that 30 percent alcohol solution in increasing amounts. At half a cup, the chronic drinker was unfazed, as "playful as ever." His companion, though, developed a slightly staggering walk and then sat down and refused to move. When they doubled the amount, even the dog accustomed to alcohol was affected: when set loose in the test chamber, his walk was a little unsteady, and he showed a preference for sitting down — although he would come when called. The other dog wove one precarious line around the room and then passed out, waking up almost twenty-five minutes later.

The two chemists repeated the comparison eleven more times, waiting a month or so between each test. The pattern never altered — ethyl alcohol visibly impaired the first-time drinker but had far less dramatic effect on the chronic imbiber. After each set of observations, the dogs were killed with illuminating gas. Samples of their brains, livers, blood, and spinal fluid were analyzed. Every time, "although the dogs were of the same weight, received the same quantity of alcohol, lived approximately the same length of time after the alcohol administration," there was less alcohol content in the organs of the habitués than in those of the novice drinkers; on average, the scientists found twice as much alcohol in their novice dogs.

To be sure, the habituated dogs showed signs of intoxication, but they did so more slowly. Once the amount of alcohol in any dog's brain climbed above 0.25 percent (+++ or more on the human scale), the animal became obviously tipsy, just as people did. This suggested something important to Gettler — that no one developed an actual immunity to the effects of alcohol. "If acquired resistance was the cause of tolerance, then the picture obtained from the analyses should be quite different," he pointed out.

If their alcohol-experienced dogs had become resistant, they should have stayed perpetually sober. If they were immune to intoxication, then those +++ brain levels should have left them unaffected. But even the most hard-headed dogs reached a point, when enough alcohol had reached their brains, that they also appeared as stumbling *drunks.*

Essentially, the Gettler and Freireich study showed how the body of a habitual drinker adjusted, became more efficient in metabolizing ethyl alcohol. The liver generated more enzymes to break the alcohol down. More liquor was processed out, so less entered the bloodstream. It thus took longer for an intoxicating amount to accumulate and reach the brain. That wasn't pure good news. Chronic drinkers needed to take in more alcohol, sometimes a lot more, to reach the level in the brain that produced intoxication. They usually responded by drinking more.

That was why experienced drinkers were credited with having such hard heads for liquor — they could drink at the same rate as their friends and be less affected. But it was not some kind of magical immunity that they acquired; rather, it was what Gettler and Freireich called the deceptively healthy, ultimately destructive internal chemistry of "the habitual drunkard."

On the first day of January 1931 the department store heir Lee Adam Gimbel jumped from the sixteenth floor of the Yale Club, having seen his fortune disappear with the economic downturn. In February the once-wealthy owner of a shoe company poisoned himself in a downtown hotel. In March a plumbing supply manager jumped from the ninth floor of the New York Athletic Club. In April the broker-husband of heiress Jessie Woolworth killed himself with mercury bichloride. In May a law firm partner dived out of his third-floor room at the Hotel Commodore, dying of a fractured skull.

The stock market, already hammered in the Black Tuesday crash of 1929, had sputtered erratically before free-falling again, pushed even deeper into trouble by economic collapses in Europe and alarming crop losses across the Great Plains states, as what appeared to be a persistent drought settled into place. During 1930 stock values had fallen a full 40 percent and two thousand banks had failed nationwide. In 1931 those numbers got worse.

In his annual report, issued that spring, Charles Norris announced that New York City had reached a new high in violent deaths the previous year — 6,525 across the five boroughs, driven by the leaping suicides that followed the economy's downward spiral. Self-terminations totaled 1,471, an average of three deaths per day. That meant that nearly one-fourth of the city's violent deaths could be attributed to despair.

Despite the bleak increase in the medical examiner's workload, the department's budget had been slashed in response to the city's own economic struggles.

"At the present time I am spending nearly $300 a month from my own personal funds for work which in my opinion has absolutely to be done to keep up the work of the office," Charles Norris wrote to the mayor's office in early 1932. "This is no pleasure to me in these depressed times, for I suffer from them just as much as anybody else. You can rest assured that I would not give out this amount of money monthly unless I considered it of importance." His department had always run on a minimal budget. But now it was less than minimal.

Gettler was doing two men's work on a salary of less than $4,000 a year; the city was refusing to fund the position of assistant chemist due to a budget shortfall, even though the salary was only $100 a month. Norris was paying a young chemist's half-time salary out of his own pocket, because "he would be down and out without it."

He was tired enough and angry enough to write a letter to the *New York Times* and complain about the mediocre administrators of a so-called great city and the difficulty of maintaining a world-class medical examiner's office: "It has been an uphill battle from the start." Norris wrote more privately to the mayor's office, announcing that he needed a vacation. He was going to spend his money on something besides subsidizing the city. He and Mrs. Norris were leaving on a steamer trip to the West Indies for a month's respite.

He would be back in late March. But if the New York City administrators hadn't learned to appreciate good forensic science by that time, he would have to reconsider whether the medical examiner's job was worth keeping.

"Altogether," Norris wrote, "the situation is becoming one where I doubt the advisability of remaining in the office permanently."

It wasn't just the budget frustrations. Norris had a depressing sense that he and other forensic scientists were trying to teach the rest of the world the same lessons, over and over again, and that the rest of the world was not really paying attention.

Harrison Martland was still trying to impress upon the rest of his profession that radium poisoning posed a public health hazard. The work had proved disheartening. He'd recently been shocked when a leading authority on industrial diseases "told me that this disease is an obscure one about which little is known.

"I cannot agree with this statement," he wrote stiffly in the introduction to a 1931 paper on the hazards of luminous paint, detailing the work done by himself, by Gettler, by physicians working for the Consumers' League, by researchers at Harvard and Yale, and by enough scientists that no one should call the problem obscure.

A steady drumbeat of dial painter deaths continued: the previous fall, Martland had logged the fifth death since the legal settlement by the New Jersey plant, a twenty-seven-year-old woman who had been bedridden at her sister's home for months after her hips crumbled. She left behind a husband and a three-year-old daughter. One of the Radium Girls from the lawsuit was also dead; another was in the hospital, her right leg having fractured as she walked across a room.

When New Jersey newspapers discovered that Martland was keeping a list of these deaths, which journalists described as "a kind of doom book," he was furious. Martland fielded dozens of calls asking whose names were in the book. He blamed the lawyers for informing the press and decided to do no further work for them. He feared that the barrage of publicity was turning the women into freaks.

"I naturally don't like to talk of it," Martland snapped to a curious reporter.

The list was intended as a record of the length of time it might take for symptoms to appear. As he'd noted in his recent paper, radium poisoning took two distinct forms. One was acute: these early deaths were characterized by severe aplastic anemia, a rapid disintegration of the bones of the jaw, spreading sores on the lips and tongue, and opportunistic bacterial infections.

The "later group," as he called it, had probably absorbed less radium at the start. Those workers sickened more slowly, gradually developing "low-grade, crippling lesions in their bones," which Martland thought were caused by the buildup of radioactive deposits in the bones themselves, followed by collapse within the bone marrow. Neither picture was a happy one. He hated the way reporters kept describing his data as a catalog of the the doomed.

"This list would hardly bring pleasant thoughts to those whose names were on it."

Norris returned from his West Indies cruise, cheered by golden weather and legal rum. On March 31, only a couple of weeks later, another radium death occurred, one that would boost the issue out of its medical backwater.

Here was an "important" radium death, the difference in response lying in the social class of the deceased. This was no Italian-American factory worker from New Jersey but a fifty-two-year-old millionaire, an industrialist, an athlete, and a member of the social elite. Eben M. Byers was chairman of A. M. Byers Iron Factory and a director of the Bank of Pittsburgh and of the Pennsylvania and Lake Erie Dock Company.

Byers had lived a life of privilege, even as the economy foundered. He was in no danger of losing his racing stables in New York, his house in Pittsburgh (where the foundry was located), or his vacation cottages in Rhode Island and South Carolina. He was a graduate of Yale, a national tennis champion, a trap shooter, and a famously fun, elegantly dressed party lover.

Five years earlier, while returning home

on a chartered train from the Harvard-Yale game, Byers had stayed up late drinking with friends. Eventually he took a drunken tumble from his sleeping berth and injured his left arm. The injury refused to completely heal. He developed an endless ache in the arm, painful enough to disrupt his sleep. He went to doctor after doctor. At length one Pittsburgh physician recommended Radithor, the radium-based health drink, sold out of Orange, New Jersey.

By the end of 1931, by his own estimate, Byers had swigged more than a thousand bottles of Radithor, never connecting the contents of the health drink with the unfortunate deaths of a few factory girls. But by that time he was also ill: his bones were mysteriously splintering, and his skin was yellowing as his kidneys failed. When he died in March 1932 in Doctors Hospital in Manhattan, he'd shrunk to a weight of ninety-two pounds. He was also exhaling radon gas.

Byers had been so secretive about his illness, so humiliated by the loss of his athletic good looks, that news of his death came as a complete shock to other businessmen. Rumors circulated that he'd lost his money, that the foundry was about to fail, that he'd poisoned himself following financial losses.

Partly to stem the panicky speculation, the city ordered an immediate autopsy from the medical examiner's office.

In fact, Mayor Walker — who was also drinking radium water to relieve his achy joints — asked Charles Norris to do the job himself. Norris sought two assistants in the work: Martland to help with the autopsy itself, and Gettler to analyze the bones.

Their report could have been taken directly from the Radium Girl case files: necrosis in both jaws, anemia, brain abscess (in the right cerebral cortex), damaged kidneys, and ravaged bone marrow, "all symptomatic of radium poisoning," Norris reported to the mayor. Byers's bones were so radioactive that when Gettler sealed them in black photographer's paper and film, he could achieve a perfect image of the dead man's vertebrae, each knobby point outlined in the rapid-fire emission of gamma and beta rays from the bone.

Only days after Norris reported the cause of Byers's death, the industrialist's influential friends were calling up their allies in Washington, D.C. The Federal Trade Commission promptly announced public hearings into the safety of drugs like Radithor, and the FDA issued a warning regarding their safety. As the *Journal of the American Medical Association* noted: "Many of the radioactive substances sold to the public for the cure of diseases are dangerous to health. Dr. Martland found that if taken as directed the amount of radioactive substance in them would be equal to that taken by dial painters in New Jersey."

At a quickly called press conference, Gettler put it more simply: "At first you feel fine. It bucks you up. Then we get ready to put parts of you in a frame." In the fall of 1932 the trade commission issued a cease-and-desist order against Bailey Radium Laboratories, which manufactured Radithor, banning transport of the material. The FDA, which had been given extremely limited authority when created in 1906 (it could do little more than warn consumers), added the Radithor case to its newly vigorous campaign for expanded legal powers. Both the United States and Europe were discussing new rules restricting all uses of radioactive materials.

And Charles Norris, caught in yet another budget fight with the mayor's office, quit his job.

The new crisis resulted from an administration change, caused by the fact that Mayor

Jimmy Walker was enmeshed in a personal scandal. His wife had divorced him over an affair with one of those pretty Ziegfeld girls, and he was under investigation for taking payoffs to help fix criminal cases. Under pressure from New York's new governor, Franklin Delano Roosevelt, who took a reform-minded approach to government, Walker had resigned in September.

An acting mayor was appointed to replace him: Joseph McKee, nicknamed Holy Joe for his purist approach. He was immediately struck by the godawful mess that Walker had made of the city budget, some of which had gone to support the silk-shirt and showgirl life the mayor had so enjoyed.

McKee found himself looking at a near $100 million deficit. The state's banks, battered by the credit crisis, refused to lend money to cover the debt. If, however, McKee could get the budget in balance, the banks were prepared to work out long-term bond financing. With everyone strapped — unemployment approaching 25 percent in the city — McKee wasn't going to consider raising taxes. So he ordered every department in the city, without exception, to cut its budget by 20 percent. That included all funding for the cars used by the medical examiner's office: the doctors would just have to catch a cab, take a train, or walk to a crime scene instead.

For Norris, who was still paying the salary of Gettler's assistant and spending his own money on equipment for autopsy rooms, it was too much. He wrote a one-sentence letter on September 19: "I herewith present my resignation as Chief Medical Examiner of the City of New York." And then he complained to everyone who would listen, which happened to include some fascinated national publications.

In his interview with *Time* magazine, Norris dwelled on his pet transportation peeve. The examiners had to be at a death scene within half an hour. They couldn't afford to spend that time on a street corner competing for cabs. "The whole thing is picayune," Norris growled to the magazine reporter. "It is easier for large departments to get a million dollars than it is for my small department to get $10. In pursuit of its penny-wise & pound-foolish policy, the city threatens to handicap seriously the work the medical examiner's office is supposed to perform."

McKee had accepted Norris's resignation "regretfully" and was shocked by the resulting furor. Thomas Gonzales was appointed acting chief for the department, but Gonzales urged the mayor to bring Norris back. So did hospitals, private physicians, university presidents, and police officers. At a ballgame between the police and fire departments, McKee took his growing dismay to the police commissioner, begging him to talk Norris into coming back. Tell him, said the mayor, that "the doctor was too valuable a public servant to lose."

As *Time* pointed out, Norris could afford to quit. He was sixty-four years old, a decent retirement age. True, he would lose his $7,500-a-year salary, but he had never done the job for the money. After all, the magazine noted, "he is one of the Pennsylvania Norrises," founders of Norristown, bankers, merchants, and landowners. He could have easily chosen comfortable relaxation.

But full-time leisure didn't suit Norris. He was happiest with a cause to fight for, a challenge to overcome. At his elegant home on West 72nd Street, he found himself missing his shabby office, the smell of blood and disinfectant in the autopsy room (he'd performed an estimated four thousand autopsies while on the job), and all his unfinished work. He grew daily more irritable and restless. When the police commissioner invited him back, Norris's wife encouraged him to return.

He moved back into the medical examiner's office in October, but only after McKee had restored car service for his department.

In November, Franklin Delano Roosevelt was elected president of the United States. The crippled economy had made Hoover and his pinched Republican policies enormously unpopular. And Roosevelt's campaign promised to alter more than financial strategies. Among his other targets was what Hoover had called "a noble experiment" and what the new president considered a failed one, the twelve-year-old constitutional amendment that had put Prohibition in place.

Many Americans believed that the alcohol restrictions had contributed to the economy's collapse, closing breweries, costing jobs, increasing crime, and — as all now admitted — increasing drunkenness. The Democratic Party had firmly backed its candidate on this issue, announcing that ending Prohibition would be one of the major aims of a new president and Congress. Roosevelt's campaign theme, "Happy Days Are Here Again," was embraced with enthusiasm; he won forty-two of the forty-eight states in the general election.

■ ■ ■ ■

At the end of 1932, Norris once again issued his holiday report on poisoned liquor deaths. The news was, for a change, unusually good. Only two people had died from methyl alcohol poisoning during the celebrations.

Norris himself had toured two neighborhoods famed for serving the city's most disreputable alcohol. One was Hoover City, along the Brooklyn waterfront, where the seamen were "known for their willingness to consume alcohol in any form." The sailors had looked encouragingly healthy. The other was the Bowery, where as usual he found grubby hallways occupied by men apparently stupefied by drinking Smoke. But "after a short nap they seemed fit enough to amble back to their favorite resorts. I guess even the Bowery speakeasies are serving a less lethal beverage." People were still poisoning themselves with ethyl alcohol; by year's end, the office had clocked in more than seven hundred deaths due to alcoholism — yet another reminder of Gettler's conclusion that ethyl alcohol might be the most important poison on their list.

But when hadn't that been true? Norris

left the Bowery in his city-financed car —
driven by his chauffeur, of course — and
returned to his office to write up his report.
It was a masterpiece of details and descriptive phrases, of falling dusk and men sleeping it off against brick walls. There was
nothing in the report that resembled the
anger with which he addressed methyl
alcohol poisonings. This was an ethyl alcohol
landscape, one that had existed long before
Norris took office and one, he suspected,
that would exist long after. He left for home
with mist gathering on the river behind him
and the cobalt sky of evening deepening to
black.

# TEN:
# CARBON MONOXIDE
# (CO), PART II
## 1933–1934

On Third Avenue in the Bronx, tucked between a small awning shop and a wedge of brick wall plastered with movie posters advertising the nearby Fenway Theater (Buster Crabbe in *Tarzan the Fearless*, Constance Bennett in *Bed of Roses*) was a dusty little store that never seemed to open for business.

But if you lived in the neighborhood, you knew that the door was unlocked at night and that behind a screen of dirty stacked boxes was a bare-bones little speakeasy, a sofa, four tables, a plywood bar along the back wall, a fair supply of whiskey, and a bartender who slept on the sofa after the bar closed.

The speakeasy, such as it was, kept its owner out of the breadlines. Barely. Sometimes his patrons paid, sometimes they didn't. They'd empty the ragtag of coins out of their pockets and put the rest on a tab.

Sometimes they paid that tab, sometimes not. The worst of the bunch was an old Irishman named Michael Malloy who drifted in and out of employment — street cleaner, coffin polisher — according to whether he was able to stay upright. Some nights the owner could have sworn that he was pouring most of his profits down Mike Malloy's skinny neck.

Malloy and money were the topics of discussion one winter night after the Irishman had passed out again atop the plywood bar. The speakeasy boss, Tony Marino, and his friends were playing an idle game of pinochle, drinking some half-decent whiskey, and worrying over the hard times. Marino's finances were borderline. The fruit vendor down the street was barely getting by, and even the local funeral home operator had a backlog of families who couldn't pay their bills. They drank some more and traded fantasies about a windfall that might save them all.

If only one of them had a wealthy relative or, barring that, a sick one with a good insurance policy. The right kind of dead family member would really have come in handy right about then. As the cards fell and the tumblers passed, the men around the table considered the idea, first as a joke, then more seriously. None of them had an expendable relative. But perhaps, Marino suggested, they could create one — someone no one would miss, someone hardly worth keeping alive.

As the story was later told, to a man, they turned to look at Mike Malloy, snoring off another bender in the backroom bar. And at that moment, in a shabby speakeasy in the Bronx, was chosen the worst possible victim for a murder scheme — a man the newspapers would later dub "Mike the Durable."

The winter of 1933 carried an icy chill, a sweep of snow across the city — and a hint that the days of speakeasies like Marino's scruffy bar were coming to an end. On February 20, Congress voted to repeal the Eighteenth Amendment. But to legally end Prohibition required that the Constitution be formally altered once again. So the legislators wrote a new amendment — the Twenty-first — which began "The Eighteenth article of amendment to the Constitution of the United States is hereby repealed."

Although both the House and the Senate approved the change, it could not become law until the new amendment was ratified by two-thirds of the forty-eight states. Because the decision remained so controversial, the federal government required that every state call a special convention to vote on ratification. Prohibition would continue as the law of the land until the Twenty-first Amendment was approved at thirty-six state convention meetings.

In the interim, the federal government had decided to loosen some of the restrictions under the Volstead Act. The first such softening was a decision permitting beer, considered a lighter alcoholic beverage, to be legally sold again. The Constitution allowed seven years for ratification. But no one expected approval of the new amendment to take very long, not even those — the dry advocates and the bootleggers — who hoped, sincerely, that it would fail.

The Mike Malloy murder conspirators numbered four: Tony Marino; his bartender, Red Murphy; the local funeral home director, Francis Pasqua; and the fruit vendor from down the street, Daniel Kriesberg. The well-connected Pasqua set up meetings with insurance agents. By the time February 1933 came around, the conspirators had wangled three life insurance policies taken on Malloy, one with Metropolitan Life for

$400 and two smaller policies with Prudential. It wasn't much money — say, by the standard set by the Snyder-Gray case — but with double indemnity for accidental death, the policies would bring in almost $1,500.

Malloy would do anything for his friends at the speakeasy — and for the unlimited drinks that Marino promised him. With no apparent suspicion, the old man signed the insurance policies, agreeing to let Pasqua pay the premium and Murphy to be named his brother and beneficiary.

Malloy was an aging wreck, maybe sixty, and homeless except when Pasqua let him sleep in the funeral home. He had the yellowed-scarecrow look of a longtime boozer. The members of the murder club figured that a mere week of unlimited alcohol would finish him off. But two weeks later, offered nightly meals of whiskey along with the sardines and crackers served as bar food, Malloy was instead thriving. He seemed to have gained a little weight and hadn't missed a personal happy hour yet.

Maybe, Marino reasoned, the problem was the liquor. Malloy was obviously well accustomed to large quantities of regular alcohol — too well, maybe. Undoubtedly he needed something stronger. Everyone knew — hadn't the medical examiner's office been preaching it for years? — that methyl alcohol made a potent drink. So Marino hurried off to acquire a supply of industrial alcohol from a gasoline station.

Red Murphy served the straight stuff to Malloy — a tumbler full on the rocks. The insurance syndicate watched the old drunk expectantly. But he didn't fall unconscious to the ground; his breathing continued with rasping regularity. He drained the tumbler and held it out for a refill. The next night he was back again. Still sucking down Marino's good liquor.

By mid-February, the conspirators gave up on alcohol poisoning.

Marino decided to kill Malloy with food instead — one of his more inventive attempts was a sandwich of rotting sardines, ground glass, and metal shavings. It failed. So did oysters marinated in wood alcohol. On an exceptionally cold night they waited until Malloy passed out, put him outside, and poured water over him. But that didn't work either: the icy water had awakened him and he'd returned to Marino's speakeasy to sleep it off on the floor.

By this time Marino had achieved a state of homicidal desperation. He brought another bar patron into the conspiracy, a cab driver named Hershy Green. He hired Green to drive over Malloy, promising that the chosen victim would be passed out and lying in the street. The payment would be $150, as soon as the insurance checks came through. The next night the conspirators lugged Malloy's unconscious body to a dark side street. Green revved the cab and the impact sent Malloy flying onto the sidewalk. They left his body for strangers to find, but in the next few days they puzzled over the lack of any newspaper story about the derelict's death.

A week later Mike Malloy limped back into the bar.

He'd been in the hospital, he told them, recovering from being hit by a car. He didn't remember it, wasn't sure how it happened. But he learned that a policeman had found him crumpled on a sidewalk and gotten him off to a hospital. He'd had a fractured skull and some broken bones, but they'd patched him back together.

Man, it still hurt though. He really could use a drink — any old bootleg variety would do.

Elsewhere, at other speakeasies, patrons were dropping dead with no problem at all.

By the end of February, nearly one hundred residents of New York were dead, killed by redistilled industrial alcohols. Brooklyn district attorney John Ruston said that the poisoned alcohol came from steamers, from rum runners in smaller boats, and as always from Brooklyn, that well-known home of creative alcohol reengineering.

"Human life must be cheap to the one who can place the dollar above it," Ruston declared. "Even if prohibition were not a law, still the distribution of such a poisonous concoction would be a crime that every law-abiding citizen should cry out to have avenged."

And by the way, he sincerely hoped that they would be soon finished with Prohibition and the murderous supply of alcohol that it had engendered. This year, if possible.

Later in February the frustrated Malloy conspirators came up with yet another murder scheme. This one would be so successful that it would mock all their earlier efforts. They would use one of the most reliable of all poisons — carbon monoxide at an unbearably high dose.

Posing as factory workers, Red Murphy and Daniel Kriesberg rented a room in a nearby boardinghouse. True, it had only a bed and no other furniture, but the room was lit by gaslight; the nozzle for the illuminating gas was right on the wall above the bed.

On the night of February 22, Murphy kept Malloy's glass full until the old man again slid unconscious to the floor. Marino, speaking loudly enough that all could hear, suggested to Murphy that he take the unconscious man home, to sleep it off. Murphy and Kriesberg then carried Malloy out the back and half-dragged, half-hauled him to the boardinghouse. The landlady, watching the trio stagger up the stairs, asked if their friend was sick. No, just drunk, they answered cheerfully.

Once they had him in bed, with the door shut, Murphy and Kriesberg worked fast. They attached a rubber hose to the gas valve and put the other end of the hose into Malloy's mouth, packing a towel over his face to close off his nostrils. Then they turned on the gas.

Malloy had withstood ethyl alcohol, methyl alcohol, rotten fish, fermented oysters, broken glass, metal slivers, an ice-water soaking, and an automobile ambush. But carbon monoxide was something else again. Later Murphy would estimate that it took less than five minutes before Malloy was dead.

Kriesberg, once he confessed, would add a little color, emulating the sound of the gas hissing like a snake as it flowed through the little rubber tube. He'd listened to it until he suddenly realized that Malloy was no longer breathing, that he could hear only the snakelike hiss of illuminating gas going into a dead man's lungs.

Toxicologists had long known that carbon monoxide killed by saturating the blood, muscling oxygen out of the way, replacing the transporter protein oxyhemoglobin with suffocating amounts of carboxyhemoglobin.

They were less sure of what made a lethal amount. The medical texts set the fatal number at somewhere between 65 and 80 percent saturation, at a minimum. But Gettler had begun to suspect that carbon monoxide might be fatal at even lower levels. The gas was such a consistent killer that it might be deadly at lower levels. Once again he decided to use his connection to the New York City morgue to test out that idea.

He tackled the job with the help of one of his favorite students, Henry Freimuth, an admired cardsharp and a first-class chemist.

They started tallying illuminating gas deaths that had come into the morgue over previous months, listing for each the carbon monoxide content of the blood at time of death:

CASE 2: Male, age 38, found dead with rubber hose leading from open gas jet to mouth. Saturation 53.6 percent.

CASE 9: Male, age 35, found dead, one gas stove jet open and not lighted; a coffee pot had boiled over and extinguished the flame. Saturation 75 percent.

CASE 50: Male, age 20, found dead in a nonventilated one-car garage. Deceased had been repairing the auto motor. Saturation 49.3 percent.

CASE 57: Female, age 40, found dead after a residence fire (fire consumed oxygen, burning material released carbon monoxide). Saturation 51.9 percent.

CASE 65: Male, age 76, found dead in bed. Coal gas had leaked from a defective flue. Saturation 61.9 percent.

Using sixty-five cases, the two scientists

found that almost 10 percent of the people in their sample had died with less than 50 percent saturation by carbon monoxide. Some had been killed by as little as 30 percent. Another 14.5 percent died with carboxyhemoglobin in the 50-to-60 percent range. More than 70 percent, as the textbooks predicted, had died after carbon monoxide reached saturation level, between 60 and 80 percent.

But it was the lower numbers that interested Gettler. They reinforced his suspicion that carbon monoxide was one of nature's most efficient killers. More than that, they illustrated one of the ongoing problems in toxicology — the difficulty of establishing a lethal dose. Some people were exceptionally vulnerable to certain poisons, while others were extraordinarily resistant.

Mike Malloy could have been, if anyone had paid attention, a case study in methyl alcohol resistance. But he would eventually come to fascinate Gettler for other reasons. How much carbon monoxide had it taken to kill such a natural survivor? And could they actually figure that out? How long did carbon monoxide saturation remain measurable in a buried corpse?

Malloy's body went into a pauper's grave

within a few days of his death.

The murder conspiracy had located a physician — a former alderman, in fact, who was willing, for another cut of the money, to sign a death certificate saying that the old drunk had died of methyl alcohol poisoning.

The funeral home director, Frank Pasqua, barely waited for the certificate to be signed before he got the body in the ground. When Metropolitan Life paid its $800 share of the insurance money, Pasqua demanded extra for the burial expenses, ignoring the obvious fact that he'd let the city bury their poison victim.

It was an unnecessary bit of cheating, a sign that things were not going to finish particularly well.

In April 1933 legal beer (3.2 percent alcohol by weight) made its triumphant, celebrated, long-awaited return.

The nation's breweries started working round the clock. One plant alone sent 350,000 cases and 18,000 kegs of beer to New York. The entire supply was consumed within two days. People bought nickel bottles by the dozen in grocery stores and from street stands. When those ran out, they bought dime bottles. Restaurants were packed with diners lingering over their gold-filled steins.

Some of the speakeasies cheerfully converted to legitimacy. They removed their concealing screens and created little beer gardens with bright-colored tablecloths and baskets of pretzels. Exuberant politicians, watching the beer flow like water, predicted that the Eighteenth Amendment would be repealed by the end of the year, buoyed by "the wet majority of a thirsty nation."

At Marino's dark little bar, though, the screen of dirty boxes stayed in place, the booze remained of the bootlegged variety, and the mood was not joyful. Not at all.

In May the Malloy murder conspiracy went to pieces.

One of Tony Marino's shady associates had been shot to death in a quarrel at the speakeasy. Bartender Red Murphy was jailed as a material witness to the murder. And Prudential Insurance had proved unexpectedly suspicious, refusing to pay its share of the death benefits. The Prudential agent was especially put off by how quickly Malloy had been buried.

Even worse, stories were starting to circulate, over card games and drinks in other Bronx bars, of the man who refused to die.

The regulars at Marino's had picked up fragments of the story and passed them on. An ever-wilder legend of the unkillable Mike floated around the shabby neighborhoods along Third Avenue. The members of the conspiracy who hadn't received their money — the cab man who'd gotten only $20 of his promised $150 — complained to their friends. The story of Mike the Durable was repeated so many times that even the beat cops heard it. One of them mentioned it to a homicide detective. After a little asking around, the detective recounted the tale to the Bronx district attorney. The prosecutor was curious enough to order an investigation.

Too many were willing to share their part of the story; too much evidence was waiting to be found. The fortunes of the murder syndicate members, such as they were, changed with the speed of a runaway elevated. On May 12 the district attorney announced that he was bringing Marino, Pasqua, Murphy, Kriesberg, and Hershy Green (the cab driver) before the Bronx grand jury. Five days and twenty witnesses later, the jury returned first-degree murder indictments against all the conspirators.

The doctor who signed the death certificate was indicted as an accessory. He pleaded guilty to failing to report a suspicious death and agreed to testify. The appalled Green accepted an assault charge — after all, he hadn't succeeded in killing Malloy — and agreed to testify in exchange for a ten-year sentence.

The others proved tougher, though. Murphy wouldn't say a word. Kriesberg suddenly decided that he wasn't sure whether or not gas had killed Mike Malloy. Marino claimed to have memory problems. The district attorney decided to delay the trial until autumn, giving himself more time to gather proof of the murder charges.

In mid-June, Bellevue Hospital and New York University announced the formation of a new department: forensic medicine. It would be the first of its kind in the country, as the dean of the university medical college put it, bringing the United States closer to the level of medical detective work done in Europe.

In fact, the term "forensic medicine" was borrowed from European institutions. The common term in the United States was "medical jurisprudence." New York University had chosen the new term both for its elite history and for its emphasis on science over law. Medical schools mostly offered a few lectures on the subject and little more. A dedicated department meant the specialty could become a credible profession. Harvard University was also starting a forensic medicine department, although that endeavor was more academic in nature. The NYU program was entirely pragmatic, focused on putting talented scientists to work in the criminal justice system.

One had only to read the list of prospective faculty to appreciate the academic expertise behind the new major — and its practical approach. Charles Norris would head the new department; Harrison Martland would be associate director. Alexander Gettler would head the toxicology section. Thomas Gonzales would teach pathology, as would most of New York City's other assistant medical examiners.

Norris had laid out an ambitious program, with training in everything from how to properly sign a death certificate to how to testify in court. An optional laboratory course, consisting of a month's work in the medical examiner's office, would give fourth-year students a chance to assist at autopsies. For newly graduated doctors who wished to do their residency in forensic medicine, the department offered a three-year practicum in the medical examiner's office, and additional postgraduate courses in toxicology.

The students would, of course, gain experiences just being on the job. The proposed curriculum didn't explain what that might entail, but in 1933 it definitely included arguing with the city's undertakers. A few enterprising funeral home directors were building business by removing bodies from crime scenes by claiming verbal permission from Norris's office. Norris had responded with a brisk memo to the police, insisting on written authorization from a medical examiner. The undertakers returned a hail of complaints about his department's unfriendly bureaucracy. One Chelsea funeral home director wrote that it had taken thirty-six hours for one family to retrieve a body from the morgue. "The clerks seem to think an undertaker is nothing and act accordingly," he wrote. "Tell those wise guys to snap out of it."

Norris apologized for any rudeness and promised to deal with it. But he didn't apologize for the new procedures. He'd discovered that some undertakers were visiting the morgue and lying about having family permission to acquire bodies. He'd ordered his clerks to release a body only after the family had verified an undertaker's claims. As Norris made clear to another irate funeral home director, he had no intention of catering to his critics:

"A great deal of the trouble really originates from the undertakers themselves. Do not imagine, however, that I am criticizing you or the Funeral Directors Association. This is merely an instance of the contrariness of the human animal."

Prohibition might still be technically the law of the land, but the country was leaving it behind.

In the month of July, according to the U.S. Brewers Association, Americans drank 1,332,790,408 glasses of freshly brewed beer. Hotel bars reopened, offering light wine as well as beer. Churches were once again permitted to use sacramental wine in services. Doctors had new flexibility in prescribing medicinal alcohol.

Repeal, once begun, gained an almost unnerving momentum. In April the first two votes, from Michigan and Wisconsin, approved the Twenty-first Amendment. In May, Rhode Island and Wyoming. In June, New Jersey, Indiana, Delaware, Massachusetts, and New York. By the end of September, twenty-five states had voted to bring back legal alcohol, meaning that ratification was two-thirds complete.

Already distributors were applying for import licenses to bring back Italian vermouth, French champagne, and Scotch whiskey. The Treasury Department felt compelled to issue public assurances that the good liquor would indeed flow when Prohibition died. "Enough Whiskey Promised Nation" read one upbeat newspaper headline, undoubtedly written by one of those alcoholic journalists who so annoyed the government's Prohibition enforcers.

Still, the illicit alcohol years had changed American culture. Gin, a new cocktail recipe, and a smoky aura had become the necessary atmosphere of any good party or hot speakeasy. The Prohibition look — drink in one hand, cigarette in the other — spoke of the new sophistication and was achieved at precious little cost.

In 1933 a pack of cigarettes cost 13 cents (two for a quarter). Carton costs averaged $1.19. Some bars set cigarettes out for free, along with sardines or, in the better speakeasies, sandwiches, cheeses, little sausages, spicy pickles, and trays of salty snacks. The cigarettes themselves came in dazzling and enticing variety, offering endless possibilities for experimentation.

Smokers could choose from among almost

three hundred brands. Cigarettes containing Turkish and Egyptian tobacco included Abdullah, Benson & Hedges, Cincinnati Club, Egyptian Straights, Hassam, Mogul, Omar, Pall Mall, Phillip Morris, Ramses, and Turkish Trophies. Blends of Turkish and American tobacco included Barking Dog, Camel, Chesterfield, Dunhill, Fatima, Lucky Strike, Marlboro, Pep, Picayune, Strollers, and Three Castles. For purists, Players and Richmond used only tobacco from Virginia and North Carolina; El Toro and Havana cigarettes were packed with leaves from the West Indies.

Cigarette smoking was so pervasive that, as Alexander Gettler discovered, the habit interfered with his research into carbon monoxide saturation of the blood.

Scientists had known since the late nineteenth century that tobacco smoke contains carbon monoxide. Victorian scientists had even been able to calculate the amount of gas in the smoke: up to 4 percent in cigarette smoke, and in Gettler's own choice of tobacco, the cigar, between 6 and 8 percent.

Gettler's latest work theorized that chain smokers might suffer from low-level carbon monoxide poisoning. He speculated in a 1933 report that "headaches experienced by heavy smokers are due in part to the inhalation of carbon monoxide." But his real interest lay less in their symptoms than in how much of the poison had accumulated in their blood, and how that might affect his calculations on cause of death.

He approached that problem in his usual, single-minded way. To get a better sense of carbon monoxide contamination from smoking tobacco, Gettler selected three groups of people to compare: persons confined to a state institution in the relatively clean air of the country; street cleaners who worked in a daily, dusty cloud of car exhaust; and heavy smokers.

As expected, carboxyhemoglobin blood levels for country dwellers averaged less than 1 percent saturation. The levels for Manhattan street cleaners were triple that amount, a solid 3 percent. But smokers came in the highest, higher than he'd expected, well above the nineteenth-century calculations. Americans were inhaling a lot more tobacco smoke than they had once done, and their saturation levels ranged from 8 to 19 percent. (The latter was from a Bronx cab driver who admitted to smoking six cigarettes on his way to Gettler's laboratory, lighting one with the stub of another as he went.)

It was safe to assume, Gettler wrote with his usual careful precision, that "tobacco smoking appreciably increases the carbon monoxide in the blood and cannot be ignored in the interpretation of laboratory results."

The other notable poison in tobacco smoke was nicotine.

Nicotine is a naturally occurring alkaloid found in tobacco plants, a tightly woven skein of carbon, hydrogen, and nitrogen ($C_{10}H_{14}N_2$). The tobacco plant, in fact, belongs to the rather notorious nightshade family, a group overpopulated with toxic vegetation, including mandrake, jimson weed, and deadly nightshade, from which the poison belladonna is produced. Nicotine had been isolated and synthesized in the nineteenth century. In pure form, it took an ounce at most to kill the average adult.

The poison is famed among toxicologists because it was the first plant alkaloid that scientists had been able to detect in a corpse. That breakthrough occurred in France in 1851, when a remarkably determined young chemist named Jean Servais Stas extracted nicotine from stomach tissues. The stomach belonged to a wealthy aristocrat who had been murdered by his financially strapped sister and her husband. Driven by evidence of the victim's suffering as he had died, the reclusive and fanatical Stas closeted himself in a laboratory until he found a way to isolate nicotine from the corpse.

In high doses, nicotine is a terrible poison — it blisters its way through tissues, burns a path from mouth to stomach, and induces intense vomiting, rapidly followed by convulsions and then a complete shutdown of the nervous system. Even in the nineteenth century, its reputation was grim. "The course of the poisoning in fatal cases is a very rapid one, measured by minutes rather than by hours," one medical textbook stated, citing one case of nicotine suicide in which the unhappy man died before he could even put the poison vial back on the table. "Death is due to respiratory paralysis," another author noted, adding that it sometimes happened so rapidly that the heart would beat on, at least briefly, after the lungs stopped working.

People had killed themselves simply by swallowing several ounces of tobacco, although that acted more slowly than the pure alkaloid. But no one was sure how much nicotine was inhaled in smoke or how dangerous it might be. For one thing, nicotine was surprisingly difficult to measure; an analysis done in 1929 pointed out that tobacco plants contained differing amounts of the poison, according to where they were grown — Virginia plants, it turned out, contained three times as much as those grown in the West Indies. And people inhaled differently as well — some puffed away rapidly, some held the smoke deep in their lungs; that would account for the range of carbon monoxide readings — from 8 to 19 percent — that Gettler had recorded when looking at smokers.

By the end of the 1920s, researchers knew that tobacco smoke contained more than nicotine and carbon monoxide. They'd also found cyanide, hydrogen sulfide, formaldehyde, ammonia, and pyridine, the latter a component in industrial solvents. A few doctors had also charted the chronic ill effects — sore throats and coughs, bronchitis, and heart and circulation problems, from rapid pulse to blocked arteries. Some even suspected that the chemistry of cigarette smoke might be linked to cancer, although that idea had plenty of skeptics.

Far more doctors argued that the beneficial effects of smoking outweighed the yet-to-be-proven risks. Tobacco chemistry seemed to stimulate the nervous system in positive ways, producing alertness but also offering a soothing effect. It helped control appetite and thereby obesity. Some physicians believed that the smoke even fended off infections through a natural antiseptic action. Doctors writing in the British medical journal *Lancet* offered the happy notion that cigarettes helped people cope with the stresses of living in the complicated world of the early twentieth century.

A comparable essay in the *Journal of the American Medical Association* cited sociability and relaxation as some of the more beneficial results of smoking tobacco. The author, while enthusiastic, acknowledged that about a third of the smokers in his own medical practice suffered from shortness of breath, a chronic cough, or both. "It still remains for the smoker to decide whether he desires to pay this price for the enjoyment he derives from it," the physician wrote.

He added an unusual note of caution. Doctors didn't understand the physiological effects of tobacco smoking, his *JAMA* editorial warned. They didn't know the entire chemical composition of the smoke. They had yet to fully realize the "the clinical effects which can be caused by it." There was reason to appreciate the habit, yes, but there was equally good reason to be wary.

In the first week of October, Marino and his friends Pasqua, Kriesberg, and Murphy at last went to trial.

During the five months since their murder indictments, the Bronx district attorney had ordered Malloy's body exhumed and sent to Bellevue for analysis. True, the old alcoholic had been underground for months, but Gettler assured the DA that if the man had been killed by illuminating gas, his laboratory would find evidence of carbon monoxide still there.

The durability of carbon monoxide in a dead body was another question Gettler fixed upon that year. German scientists had reported, two years earlier, that bodies exhumed after three months in the ground still contained carboxyhemoglobin. Was that its limit? Gettler wondered. Or was the compound even longer-lasting?

He'd filled sixteen bottles with blood from people, including Malloy, who had died of CO poisoning. All the blood samples were saturated with carboxyhemoglobin. Half of them had gone into the lab icebox and half onto one of the long wooden shelves that lined the laboratory wall. His idea was simply to compare the cells' rate of decay in cold preservation conditions versus room temperature. Gettler and his staff checked the bottles at intervals ranging from twenty-four hours to eighty-four days after first storage. "In no case was the carbon monoxide increased by putrefaction," he'd noted, reaffirming the fact that after death a human body neither made nor absorbed the gas.

Gettler found that carboxyhemoglobin did diminish as the blood cells decayed. But its disappearance was slow, barely detectable in the earliest measurements. At the longest interval, eighty-four days, the carbon monoxide saturation declined only from 75.3 to 70.8 percent, a fatal reading at either amount. And Mike Malloy's blood? His CO saturation measured at that still potent 70 percent. Equally damning, on autopsy, the old man's heart and lungs were stained bright with the all too familiar cherry red.

On October 19, 1933, all four plotters were found guilty of first-degree murder. The following day they were sentenced to die in the electric chair, the date to be set pending appeal, and depending on how soon the conspirators could be fitted into the schedule at Sing Sing.

In Manhattan, as the clock ticked away on

the end of the hated Prohibition years, the mood at the city's hotels, clubs, and restaurants was a feverish mix of anticipation and celebration.

The Waldorf-Astoria outfitted three new bars, two small and cozy, and one, off the hotel's admired Peacock Alley, to outshine all others with its blue mirrored ceiling, silver-shell walls, and gleaming blue and gold columns. The Hotel New Yorker bought $100,000 worth of good whiskey and was in the process of building a subbasement wine cellar, an indoor bar, and an elegant outdoor terrace restaurant.

The Yale Club, the Harvard Club, and the Racquet Club had all filed to reopen their bars. By late November, requests for liquor licenses were coming into New York's city hall at the rate of one thousand a day, and nationally, the government was permitting alcohol production at such a rate that 125 million gallons were expected to be available as soon as the dry era officially ended.

By the end of November thirty-three states had voted for repeal and, three more — Ohio, Pennsylvania, and Utah — had scheduled votes on December 5. The master chef of the Hotel Pierre predicted a return to fine dining, elegant dancing and an end to the "restless jazz and hip flask" days of

Prohibition. The chef had real hope, he confided to a sympathetic newshound, that men and women might linger over their wine rather than dancing around the tables while they awaited their food.

The manager of Louis Sherry's, the stylish two-story restaurant at 300 Park Avenue, worried that customers would have to relearn the appropriate wine for each course. He wasn't even sure his waiters remembered — all anyone knew anymore was bathtub gin and renatured alcohol. The kitchen at Sherry's was planning a new menu: caviar with vodka, terrapin with sauterne, pressed duck with champagne (preferably Cliquot Brut 1921), and an after-dinner drink of café brulé (hot coffee, cognac, and a cinnamon stick, served in a glass with a sugared rim).

"It means the end of drunkenness," the Sherry doorman predicted. "We won't search the place after a party to find the boys and girls who have slid under the tables. We're heading back to the days of fine manners. I feel it in my bones."

Utah, the last state needed to complete ratification, did so at exactly 5:33 p.m. Eastern Time on December 5. States like New York found that timing wholly irritating. Repeal came so late in the day that most retail liquor stores — a good five thousand now had licenses — were unable to get their newly legal stock into the city that night.

Still, the well-prepared hotels rolled out bar carts, wheeling them through the lobbies to dispense cocktails. Bloomingdale's department store had been savvy enough to acquire its own liquor permit, and the moment the radio flashed news of the Utah vote, it sold waiting customers bottles of imported scotch and rye.

The line at Bloomingdale's snaked out the door and into the noisy, shouting, jubilant streets.

There was other change to celebrate. After fifteen years of Tammany Hall control, after the scandalous departure of Gentleman Jimmy Walker, the city of New York finally had elected another reform mayor. Unfortunately, Charles Norris didn't get along with Fiorello H. La Guardia any better than he had with previous city leaders.

La Guardia, elected in November, promptly began dealing with the city's still appalling deficit ($31 million). He trimmed salaries, laid off city employees, and raised fees. And in January 1934 he'd ordered all the fat trimmed from departmental budgets. La Guardia's enthusiastic staffers even removed what they saw as an overabundance of timepieces, including the wall clock at the medical examiner's office.

Norris immediately paid for a replacement clock himself, but he was infuriated enough to once again complain to the city papers, regardless of whether it embarrassed La Guardia.

It wasn't a matter of fat, Norris snapped: "For years our budget has been cut to the bone. Now the bone is being scraped." Didn't the mayor's office know anything about how a medical examiner's office had to operate? "The law requires that we record the exact time a case is reported to us and the staff is dependent on that clock for accuracy. Enough said for such economy."

Mayors, he'd learned, had to be trained to appreciate the science of forensic medicine. Repeatedly.

On June 3, 1934, Tony Marino, Frank Pasqua, and Daniel Kriesberg went to the electric chair. Their fellow conspirator, Red Murphy, had won a two-week stay while the courts evaluated his mental status. The three men said good-bye to their families, met with their spiritual advisers, and waited in the Dance House for the call to execution.

A reporter for the *New York Daily Mirror* recorded the events in the crisp staccato of a machine gun: "It's 11 o'clock," wrote the *Mirror*'s Robert Campbell. "The crack of doom. Now the flic-flac of feet. The unlocking of the door." The prisoners' march down the so-called Last Mile, really only about two dozen steps. Pasqua went first: "The kw-e-e- of the dynamo. Two thousand volts and ten amperes. The rip-saw current that tears one apart. Three shocks." Next Marino. Another three shocks. Then Kriesberg. Three shocks again. All the three men were dead in seventeen minutes. Just over a month later, having lost that last appeal, Red Murphy, angrily unrepentant, went to the electric chair as well.

Campbell summed it all up — the shrill song of the dynamo, the dark fire of the electric current, the rumble of bodies wheeled away on the stone floor, all in the terms of a newly liberated lover of whiskey: "It's the State's toast to old 'Mike the Durable.' "

# Eleven:
# Thallium (Tl)
## 1935–1936

There were times, and they came frequently enough, when one could believe that modern society, machine-age America, was addicted to poisons. Every day retold the story of that dependency: poisons floated in the exhaust-smudged air of the morning commute and swam in the evening martini, in the gas-fed blue flames of the stove, in the soft smoke of the after-dinner cigarette, in the barbiturates that so many now swallowed at the end of a stressful day.

In a best-selling book, *100,000,000 Guinea Pigs* (reprinted nine times by 1935), a pair of consumer-advocate authors complained that American citizens had become test animals for chemical industries that were indifferent to their customers' well-being. The government, they added bitterly, was complicit. Regulation was almost nonexistent. The nineteen-year-old FDA was a joke, lacking authority to set even minimal

418

safety standards. For two years consumer groups and their allies in Congress had been trying — unsuccessfully — to get a new law passed that would give the FDA meaningful authority.

Their demands were not particularly extravagant. The proposed legislation would require safety testing before a product was introduced on the market. It would establish corporate liability for marketing hazardous products. One of the proposals — fought by an unholy alliance of industrial manufacturers and patent medicine companies — simply required that consumers be provided with basic information, for instance that ingredients be listed on containers of medicine, household cleaners, and cosmetics.

In 1935 a woman seeking to darken her lashes with Lash Lure had no way of knowing that the dye contained a benzene compound that could — and did — cause corneal ulcers and blindness. A balding man using Acme Hair Rejuvenator had no way to know he was rubbing lead acetate into his scalp. Stillman's Freckle Remover was loaded with mercury, according to medical tests. A popular coloring agent, Mrs. Potter's Walnut Tint Hair Stain, advertised itself as "guaranteed free from lead, sulfur, and silver" but contained an aniline dye, derived from coal tar, that was banned in Europe because of its toxic properties. In the United States, of course, federal agencies had no power to take such protective actions.

The authors of *100,000,000 Guinea Pigs,* Arthur Kallet and F. J. Schlink of the Consumer's Research Union, devoted a large section of their book to a worst-case cosmetic: depilatory creams that contained the metallic element thallium. It was no secret that thallium was poisonous; it was the main ingredient in a number of pesticides. Yet cosmetics makers used it anyway, insisting that it was safe in small doses and advertising its amazing ability to remove unwanted hair from the face — and anywhere else on the body that a woman might desire.

The depilatory creams had created a small but significant epidemic in the early 1930s, fully recounted in the *Journal of the American Medical Association.* A woman had applied the cream to her chin and ended up almost completely bald, barring about one hundred hairs forming "a fringe on the back of her neck." A woman in Minnesota had used the cream on her upper lip and ended up hospitalized, her hair coming out in clumps, her legs unable to support her. A woman in Maine had lost her vision. "Could there be lead in the cream?" her doctor wrote to ask AMA experts, saying that her other symptoms — including severe nausea — reminded him of acute lead poisoning, which could cause the corneas to become opaque.

Kallet and Schlink issued repeated warnings against thallium-based creams, which they said were, of all poisons, "one of the most deadly known," and urged consumers to lobby their congressmen for better regulation of such compounds. The AMA had been campaigning against such products for years. Due to the lack of government regulation, it had created its own Bureau of Investigation, which analyzed numerous brands and warned repeatedly that thallium creams were a "menace to public health."

But women bought the beauty products anyway. Women's magazines, such as *Vogue,* carried advertisements extolling the potions' ability to remove unsightly hair and lend a beautiful pale luster to skin. After all, these ubiquitous poisons worked as advertised. Tetraeythyl lead did solve engine knocks; carbon monoxide did provide an inexpensive and reliable fuel; cyanide did help neatly fix clear photographic images on film.

And thallium, as promised, did cause hair to painlessly fall out, did make it disappear like snow on an unexpectedly warm morning.

April that year of 1935 blew in gold, with hints of summer: crowds packed the boardwalks at Coney Island during the day and sunned the afternoons away on Long Island beaches. Not that Frederick Gross could afford a beach trip, but sunshine was free. In the gentle light of evening, he liked to sit with neighbors on the high stoop of his rooming house, smoke a pipe, and trade stories about the day, watching the kids play kick-the-can in the street.

He was such a nice man, his neighbors said. He never complained about being a cripple; he just gave himself a little extra time because he moved so slowly with his artificial leg. His right leg had been amputated below the knee following a carriage accident in his native Philadelphia. He'd worked for thirteen years as a bookkeeper at an importing firm in lower Manhattan. His co-workers liked him too. He was kind-natured, they said, hardworking, friendly in his quiet way.

Gross, his wife, Barbara, their five children, and his mother-in-law lived in a small cold-water flat in Brooklyn's Bushwick neighborhood, where the streets were lined with houses that had been divided and then divided again into rooms for rent. Their next-door neighbor swore that the walls were so thin she could hear every word spoken in the Gross household. She'd never heard him raise his voice in anger, she told the police.

Yes, the neighbor said, it was true that by the end of April his wife and four of his children were dead. Yes, the remaining son and mother-in-law were both hospitalized. But she would never, never believe that the little bookkeeper with the sweet smile had killed them all.

The first sign that things were about to go wrong — terribly, unbelievably wrong — for the Gross family came on an ordinary day in late March. When Gross returned home for dinner, his wife, Barbara, told him that one of the boys didn't feel well.

Nine-year-old boys like Freddy were always picking up colds and stomach upsets. Gross put his eldest son into pajamas and tucked him into bed. The boy seemed pale, though. Gross decided to stay in the room in case his son got worse. He was dozing in the chair when Freddy suddenly woke up retching and gasping for breath. By early morning the child was dead. And then the next day their three-year-old, Leo, fell ill. He died the first week of April.

Their doctor reported both deaths to the Department of Health as bronchial pneumonia. But by that time Barbara Gross was also desperately ill. She died two days after little Leo, on April 4. This time the hospital doctors diagnosed the cause as encephalitis. Stunned, Gross requested a few days off work. He and his mother-in-law worked together to care for the remaining children, seven-year-old Katherine, five-year-old Frank, and the baby of the family, Barbara, who was eighteen months old.

Curiously, only the father seemed healthy. The rest of them dragged; even the usually energetic youngsters were tired and a little achy. Gross's sister-in-law started coming by almost daily, helping with dinner, letting her children play with the Gross youngsters. But things only got worse.

By the end of the month both the little girls were dead, diagnosed with encephalitis, and the grandmother and the five-year-old were in the hospital. And all four of them, the dead and the sick, were almost completely bald. The neighbors had been wondering about it for weeks. The youngest, Barbara, had once had the most beautiful head of curly brown hair. Her mother had

424

been so proud of it that she'd showed the little girl off up and down Eldert Street, where they lived. But by mid-April the toddler's hair was so thin that her scalp showed through, and two days before the little girl died, one neighbor said, "She was as bald as your hand."

The name *thallium* comes from the Greek word *thallos* for a newly leafed plant, brilliant with the sun-bright green of spring. It seems a strangely vivid description for a less-than-colorful metallic element, silvery pale in the ground, darkening to tarnished gray when exposed to air.

But the story of its scientific discovery explains the name, as well as the scientific advances entailed in that discovery. Thallium was first identified in 1861 by a leading British chemist. William Crookes had been asked to analyze a batch of sulfuric acid, used in industrial mining, which was apparently tainted with an unknown impurity. Following his usual routine, Crookes started with a simple flame test. He dipped a platinum wire into the acid and put the wire into the colorless fire of a Bunsen burner.

As it heated, the wire lit to a sudden brilliant green.

Crookes had done hundreds of flame tests. He'd seen other elements that flashed green — copper and barium, for example. But the springlike exuberance of this color was new to him. He decided to run a more sophisticated test on a new instrument, the spectroscope. The device worked on the same principle as the flame test: when a material heats to incandescence, it emits light of varying colors according to its atomic makeup. In a spectroscope, an unknown compound was heated until it glowed. The resulting light was directed through a slit and into a prism. The prism then refracted the light into its full spectrum, whatever that might be. A scientist looking at those bright shimmers through a magnifying tube could identify each component of the heated material, matching the color to the existing chemical catalog.

But the clear green line that Crookes saw in the spectroscope was unknown, leading him to realize that he'd found a new element. He named his discovery thallium, for its unique spectroscopic color. As it turned out, Crookes would be forced to share the credit. That same year, a chemist in France, Claude-August Lamy, reported finding surprising green lines of light in tests of mining residues. Lamy had taken the discovery further, isolating the element and casting a small metallic ingot. The French scientist also (although this would be appreciated only much later) provided the first suspicions that thallium was a treacherous material.

During the months that he spent isolating thallium, Lamy's health progressively faltered. He suffered from a stumbling exhaustion and shooting pains in his legs. He recovered, but he was troubled enough to further test the element by feeding it to dogs, ducks, and chickens. All died in a few days, suffering from weakness, trembling, difficulty breathing, and, in the worst instance, paralysis in their legs.

Crookes greatly resented what he saw as an attempt to steal his discovery, and he refused to accept his rival's concerns. At high doses thallium might be dangerous, the British chemist acknowledged. But small doses, which he'd tried himself, had no health effects at all.

Crookes edited a leading chemistry journal, so his well-publicized assessment was the one that gained scientific acceptance. It was too bad, of course, that in this particular detail he was wrong.

"Five in Family Killed by Rare Poison" read

the *New York Times* headline on May 11. The Gross family story rated the newspaper's front page; after all, how often did a $ 20-a-week clerk, as the paper put it, murder his own children with an exotically unusual toxic agent?

The deaths had been too many, and too close together, to avoid investigation. The police work started after Gross's last remaining child, little Frank, and his mother-in-law, Olga Bein, ended up in Brooklyn's Bushwick Hospital. A local physician, who had just acquired a spectroscope, was sent tissue scrapings taken in the hospital. The tests resulted in an unmistakable evil dazzle of green. The district attorney then had the bodies of Gross's wife and eldest son exhumed. In those tests as well, the physician saw the lethal green signature of thallium.

The police questioned Gross for twenty-eight frustrating hours, trying to get him to confess to the murders. He maintained his innocence and bewilderment — he could not understand how thallium had been found in the bodies of his family. By the time he was sent to his jail cell, he sat down on the cot and fell straight asleep, still dressed in his one good suit.

Thallium was surprisingly easy to obtain,

despite what Alexander Gettler described as "its relatively rare occurrence and high cost." Beyond its cosmetic uses, it had been incorporated into a wide array of industrial products.

Thallium served to strengthen the filaments in tungsten lamps. When metallic thallium was melded into glass, it strengthened light refraction, making it valuable in manufacturing eyeglass lenses and in giving sparkle to artificial gemstones. Added to the mercury alloy used in thermometers, thallium helped achieve accuracy down to minus 60 degrees centigrade.

Concentrated doses of thallium salts were used in pest control; it had been mixed into rodent poisons since 1920, sold as Zelio paste and Thalrat. It was the toxic ingredient in a pest-killing bait marketed as Thalgrain. In the early twentieth century it had been used to remove the hair of children with scalp infections, such as ringworm, so that doctors could see and treat the fungus. But that practice had been abandoned when too many of the toddlers died.

As the U.S. Public Health Service noted in a review of thallium's use in medicine, every animal tested — mice, rats, guinea pigs, dogs, rabbits, and apes — lost its hair or fur when taking a daily dose of thallium.

Researchers were unsure exactly why. That thallium was the only metallic poison to cause loss of hair seemed peculiar, but animal research suggested that it was related to an unusually rapid destruction of skin cells. Later studies would find that one reason thallium caused such accelerated damage was that it possesses an atomic structure very like another soft metal, potassium. In the same way that radium takes advantage of the body's natural affinity for calcium, thallium tends to move rapidly along potassium-uptake channels into the nuclei of cells.

But where potassium helps maintain a proper fluid balance in cell walls and feeds the nerve cells that control muscle movement, thallium disrupts cell metabolism and splinters apart chemical bonds. The potassium channels too provided a depressingly efficient way to spread the poison's effects. "Animals poisoned with thallium, that have been examined after death, showed the metal to be present in almost every tissue in the body," wrote one government scientist, arguing that the element was so indiscriminately lethal that it shouldn't even be used as a pesticide.

For several years, starting in the late

1920s, the State of California had used grain poisoned with thallium bait to eradicate ground squirrels in its southern coastal counties. As state wildlife officials discovered, the plan worked, except that it also killed animals that ate the poisoned squirrels — civets, coyotes, weasels, foxes, red-tailed hawks, golden eagles, turkey vultures — as well as any creature unfortunate enough to find leftover bait, which included mourning doves, quail, rabbits, pheasants, five species of wild geese, meadowlarks, skunks, rats, ravens, three species of sparrow, three species of woodpecker, kangaroo rats, juncos, white-footed mice, pet cats and dogs, domestic chickens, sheep, and cows.

The program was finally discontinued after a group of field workers used a sack of grain found in a grower's barn to make dinner. It turned out to be a sack of thallium bait. Seven of the workers died, and more than a dozen others survived but suffered partial paralysis and, of course, the telltale, inescapable hair loss.

The Gross tragedy spurred Gettler to conduct a detailed analysis of thallium toxicology. He concluded that about a third of an ounce of thallium salts would quickly kill just about anyone.

The symptoms of a concentrated dose, he wrote, were nausea and vomiting, trembling, shortness of breath, and collapse into death within about thirty hours. In fact, such symptoms were not so different from those of a virulent pneumonia, which was exactly the diagnosis of the two Gross boys to die most quickly. "In subacute cases, where the patient lives for several days to three or four weeks," Gettler wrote, "the only characteristic sign is alopecia (hair loss) but only in those cases where death was delayed for at least 20 days."

In these gradual poisonings, the first indications were varied: nausea, diarrhea, pain in the legs, tremors, paralysis, "symptoms and signs simulating encephalitis, occasionally with psychotic manifestations such as mental depression or excitation, delirium and dementia, convulsions, coma and death due to paralysis of the central nervous system and respiratory failure." These symptoms too could be easily mistaken for an infectious disease or sometimes a state of neurosis — and often were. In a famous murder case, a woman in Austria killed two husbands, her son, and a baby daughter with thallium between 1924 and 1934. She was caught only after she started killing lodgers in her rooming house. And that wasn't because police suspected her; rather, the son of a formerly healthy lodger insisted that his mother's body be exhumed, leading to an exposure of the murders.

Thallium is colorless, odorless, and tasteless. It mixes easily into liquids, without the occasional grittiness of arsenic. It can be disguised by almost any beverage — coffee, tea, soda, and cocoa. The police investigation found that Gross's employer had recently acquired a small shipment of cocoa with the idea of adding it to the distribution list. After rejecting that idea, the company had offered the cocoa to employees at twenty cents a can. Frederick Gross had purchased four half-pound tins of cocoa shortly before his family started dying.

Surely, the Brooklyn detectives thought, that was more than he needed. It seemed he'd been planning to practically force-feed his family cocoa. Further investigation found that the import firm kept a supply of thallium sulfate on hand to keep down the building's rodent population. The police sent one of the cocoa tins left in the Grosses' flat to the doctor they'd been using in the investigation.

Once again he reported back that when he put the sample into the spectroscope, he saw that unmistakable, undeniable warning flash of green.

"So far we have uncovered nothing that would indicate a motive except poverty," the Brooklyn district attorney announced, but the poverty was severe: "The man had a hard time of it."

Frederick Gross had never made much money, but the Depression had sent his finances skidding to near destitution. By 1934 his employer, the importing firm Pfaltz & Bauer, had lost so much business that it had given staffers a choice of taking a pay cut or being let go. Gross's salary had been cut from $35 a week to $20.

The family apartment — cold water, without light or heat — cost $20 a month. That left the Grosses barely $15 a week for all other expenses. They'd taken to eating hot cereal at every meal. That was why he bought the cocoa, Gross said — it was sweet and filling. They'd had it with dinner every night — a bowl of hot farina with a little milk and sugar, and a cup of steaming cocoa. His wife often gave it to the children with lunch as well — cocoa, cereal, and a little orange juice on good days.

Even so the family was sinking into debt. Gross owned one suit — a blue serge, which he was paying off on an installment plan.

On the day he was arrested, he still owed $17 out of the $30 that the suit had originally cost. The family was two months behind on rent; in April the Grosses had learned that another child was on the way. "All of it might just have been too much for him. That might have been the motive."

The reporters picked up on the note of uncertainty in that statement. It wasn't just Gross's dogged insistence of innocence that caused the uncertainty. The police had found no evidence that he'd purchased or stolen the poison. No one had seen him mixing anything into the cocoa. In fact, he usually left meal preparation to his wife and mother-in-law. There was nothing to say that he had benefited from the deaths. He'd taken out no helpful life insurance policies.

Even more telling, the detectives hadn't identified a single person who believed in his guilt. Usually, it was easy enough to find someone who'd claim that they'd always suspected the accused. But this time none of the neighbors did — none of the family or friends. His mother-in-law, still in the hospital recovering from thallium poisoning, told the police that she simply didn't believe it. His sister-in-law said the same. Gross didn't have a mean bone in his body, she insisted to the police, and had loved his family.

"I am confident that the mystery surrounding the deaths will be cleared up," the Brooklyn district attorney, William Geoghan, told reporters. "Any possibility of an accident has already been excluded." But privately he was less confident. He decided to seek the opinion of someone besides the local physician. He sent the evidence — body tissues, cocoa, the works — to the city laboratories at Bellevue.

In cases of thallium poisoning, autopsy results can be frustrating.

The element creates no characteristic damage, nothing like the gaudy red signal of carbon monoxide, or the bone-splintering evidence of radium poisoning. In cases of acute thallium poisoning, Bellevue pathologists found, the bodies showed perhaps an inflammation of the stomach lining, a few bloody patches in the organs, but nothing that wasn't found in a host of other conditions as well.

Thallium doses that killed more slowly, of course, usually produced hair loss. But again, internally the poison provided nothing in the way of dramatic evidence. There might be signs of clotting in the blood vessels, fatty degeneration in the heart and kidneys, congested lungs, or an excess of blood in the brain. But two of the Gross children had been exhumed and autopsied, and in both cases "the findings were entirely negative."

It all added up to another reason that thallium deaths were so easily and often mistaken for other causes. Only in the laboratory did thallium give itself away. In the manner of other metallic poisons, such as arsenic, thallium lodges stubbornly in the body, permeating the tissues for weeks and even months after death. Any knowledgeable forensic toxicologist can find it there.

It is, one might say, a chemist's poison.

Like the Brooklyn physician, Gettler ran a spectroscopic analysis of the tissues and the cocoa. He also saw the green flash of light with each sample. But one test wasn't enough for him. It never was.

He went on to use a spectrograph, a piece of equipment similar to a spectroscope but with a camera to make permanent images of the lines of light. He'd found spectrographic images extremely useful in court testimony. These "photographic flashes," as he called them, also revealed thallium in every sample of tissue.

The spectrographic lines from the cocoa, however, he found less convincing — the color seemed off to him. And the cocoa had turned a little rancid — Gettler wondered if it could have leached some metal from the can itself. He suspected the alloy used to make the container included some copper, which could account for the greenish glow of the cocoa results.

He decided to run a series of chemical tests on both the cocoa and the tissue — an old-fashioned technique, compared to the new machinery, but reliable. He repeated the tests, to his satisfaction, over a period of four days.

While Gettler was running those tests, the police began discussing an entirely different theory to explain the murders.

In their search of the Eldert Street apartment, Brooklyn police officers had found several books with Mrs. Gross's name on the flyleaf. Two were medical books, with information on different poisons. The last was philosopher Arthur Schopenhauer's *Studies in Pessimism,* which despairingly contends that at core, the universe offers no hope of a rational existence.

Geoghan, the district attorney, at first dismissed the books as unimportant, but then neighbors filed in with stories about Mrs. Gross. A woman who lived two doors down made and signed a statement about a conversation she'd had several weeks before the chain of deaths began. Mrs. Gross — after learning that she was pregnant again — had said that she intended to kill her children, her mother, and herself with rat poison.

She told the neighbor that she already had the poison and that it was slow, painless, and sure to kill. "Do you mean you'd give your children poison and see them suffer?" the horrified friend asked. She said that Mrs. Gross replied: "There's no suffering to what I've got. It's sure death." She'd learned about the poison when she worked as a telephone operator in a Philadelphia hospital. "It may take a day. It may take thirty days." She just couldn't bear to raise her children in such desperate poverty.

But, her friend told the police, Mrs. Gross didn't want to poison her husband. Without the expense of a large family, she was sure he'd find a better life. According to the statement, she'd declared: "I have the best husband any woman could want. But rather than drudge along like this and live in poverty I'd do anything."

The strongest objection to that theory of

the crimes came from Frederick Gross, still in jail. He and Barbara had been married twenty years, since they'd met in Philadelphia. She was good woman and a good mother, he told the police. "It could never have happened that way," he told the district attorney. "I don't believe it."

But the neighbors kept telling their stories, and even the prosecutor was starting to wonder.

The chemical tests for thallium were an intricate, delicate business.

First, Gettler ground the tissue into slush. Then he poured in some nitric acid and let the mixture stand in a large flask for an hour. Then the flask went into a steam bath for two hours until all the tissue was completely dissolved. The solution was cooled, any solidified fat was filtered off through glass wool, and the flask was placed over an open flame. As the liquid heated, sulfuric acid was poured carefully into it.

Once the acid boiled off, a thick sludge remain to bubble blackly over the burner. "It is well to lower the flame at this point, and then to increase it again when the charred liquid has quit frothing," Gettler recommended in a paper detailing his methods. After the liquid settled down, he trickled nitric acid into the mix, slowly, until the color changed from black to red to yellow and finally to a colorless state of clarity. Only then, after other contaminants had been ruthlessly removed, would he begin to check for thallium.

The poison could be found by several methods. One was that old standard, the flame test. The others involved forcing thallium to settle out of the solution. For instance, if sulfur dioxide was bubbled through the clear liquid and a hydrogen solution added, a pale-yellow, thallium-rich layer would settle to the bottom of the flask. Or one could add an iodine compound and precipitate out thallous iodide. Ammonia and potassium chromate caused a bright-yellow layer to coat the bottom, consisting of thallous chromate.

Of course, negative results were equally easy to see. If there was no thallium in the mixture, the liquid in the flask remained innocently transparent. To Gettler's surprise, he ended up with both results — the sullen yellows of thallium, and the rainwater clarity of a poison-free solution.

The chemical tests run by Gettler's laboratory found thallium in all the dead children, but not in the body of Mrs. Gross. She had apparently died of encephalitis, as originally diagnosed. The children had been poisoned, but the mother not at all, providing yet another theory — that she was somehow deranged enough to want to start her marriage over, with only her husband and the single child yet to come.

Gettler's results showed that each child had received a markedly different dose of thallium. Because the two girls had died after their mother, the district attorney was convinced that their father had to be the poisoner. But Gettler disagreed. Partly because the children had been going bald in the weeks before their deaths, he thought they'd received the poison before the mother died, killed more slowly by a lower dose than the two boys got.

Further, repeated analyses of the cocoa found not a trace of thallium sulfate, the rat poison used by Gross's employer. If the can had contained poison, Gettler pointed out, they should have found it at greater levels than in the decomposing tissues. Based on Gettler's findings, the autopsies, and other pathology work done at Bellevue, the medical examiner's report proposed that while the children had been poisoned by thallium, there was no evidence linking the deaths to the father.

The Brooklyn authorities, and especially the doctor who had done the original tests, were taken aback. The doctor, even more, was angrily embarrassed. Perhaps, he suggested, Gettler wasn't used to the spectroscope. Everyone made mistakes, even New York City's apparently infallible toxicologist. He publically recommended that Gettler try the tests again.

That prompted Charles Norris, who brooked no criticism of his hardworking and underpaid staff, to intervene. If Alexander Gettler failed to find any trace of the poison, Norris stated, then "it was not there." Period.

On May 20, a Brooklyn magistrate dismissed the charges against Frederick Gross. His employer called the newly released bookkeeper to tell him that they'd held the job for him. Gross went straight to the hospital where his son, Frank, was in bed on a sun porch. Seeing the little bald boy in the crib, he started to cry. The five-year-old asked his father why he hadn't come to see him on visiting Sundays.

"I was busy, son," Gross replied. He told reporters that when his son was well enough, he was going to take him to a summer camp to play and get stronger. His mother-in-law had agreed to keep house for him again. He hoped to do a better job of taking care of his remaining family.

And so, as soon as possible, he was going back to work. He didn't blame the district attorney, he said. He knew things had looked bad. But he had one special request of the journalists who gathered around to hear his plans: just tell everyone, just spread the word, that he had been innocent all along.

"Let your voice be heard loudly and often in protest against the indifference, ignorance and avarice" responsible for causing poisonous compounds to so permeate everyday life, wrote Kallet and Schlink of the Consumers' Research Union in the 1935 edition of their manifesto. "In adulteration and misrepresentation lurks a menace to your health that ought no longer be tolerated."

The CRU was starting to wonder what poisoning issue would stir the government into taking action. The FDA had sidestepped Ginger Jake, turning that investigation over to the Treasury Department's Prohibition enforcement officers. Although the agency had taken steps to end the use of radium-laced health waters such as Radithor, there were still no laws that prohibited interstate commerce in such risky products. Neither had Congress strengthened the FDA in response. Instead, legislators and even President Roosevelt were resisting such laws, on the grounds that they would be detrimental to business at a time of economic crisis.

The CRU feared it would take a catastrophe to change the system. In that assessment Kallet, Schlink, and their colleagues would be proved right two years later. In 1937 a small Tennessee pharmaceutical company developed a new kind of cough syrup by dissolving a sulfa drug into the solvent diethylene glycol — a complex chain of carbon, hydrogen, and oxygen ($HO-CH_2-CH_2-O-CH_2-CH_2-OH$) also used in antifreeze formulas. Diethylene glycol had a sweet taste to it anyway, but the company made the elixir even better-tasting by adding raspberry flavoring.

That product, Elixir Sulfanilamide, killed more than one hundred people, most of them children. Under the FDA's minimal rules, though, the company was required to pay only a small fine for mislabeling, because "elixirs" were supposed to contain alcohol and this formula had none. The deaths spurred a consensus of outrage, led by the grieving families and intensified by the furious consumer advocates and the anguished physicians who had killed their patients. (As one wrote, he'd watched his own friends die as a result of asking him to treat them.) The head of the company stoked the national anger further by pointing out that barring the mislabeling, the product had been entirely legal: "I do not feel that there was any responsibility on our part."

The following year Congress passed and Roosevelt signed the 1938 Food, Drug and Cosmetic Act, which empowered the FDA to demand safety testing and accurate labeling and to hold manufacturers legally responsible for harming their customers.

That spring of 1935, despite the successful resolution of the Gross case, Charles Norris just felt tired. Another poison. Another murder. Another series of unnecessary deaths. Another story to break your heart.

That April, for the first time in years, he did not attend the Detectives' Endowment Association's annual party at the Hotel Astor ("I am avoiding going out as much as possible") and simply sent a contribution. When his alma mater, Yale, asked for a donation to the alumni fund, he wrote back candidly to the old friend leading the drive:

"You ask me how I am. I am just recovering from a bad attack of the 'flu.' We must remember that we are all getting old and tired, and my expense account is much larger than my income and it has been so for some time."

He promised to send a check for fifty dollars, but only in May, when he was sure it would clear. He was putting his spare money into the medical examiner's office and his spare time into dealing with Mayor La Guardia, who seemed to believe that all longtime department heads must be crooks. La Guardia had ordered examinations of all such departments, and in late May the mayor's political allies, organized into a Citizens' Budget Committee, charged Norris's staff with pocketing illegal fees for routine work such as issuing death certificates.

The commission calculated that 40 percent of the cases handled by Norris's office required some sort of certified paperwork. That meant more than 20,000 potentially moneymaking opportunities over the previous seventeen years. At worst, if the medical examiner's office charged $20 per report — a fee that had been set by other departments — then the graft total would approach $400,000 since Norris took office.

Norris called the report a joke: "I don't know where they get any estimates of $400,000. The insurance companies occasionally want copies of the hearings, and they pay small fees for them, but we don't get those requests at the rate of more than two a week and the fee runs from fifty cents to a dollar." And poor people, he added, had always been given paperwork at no cost at all.

Within a month a formal investigation by the city's commissioner of accounts had cleared Norris's office of graft charges. True, the office charged typing fees for lengthy documents, but they ran about fifty cents. The employees apparently had considered this a practice allowed under the law. They did it openly. Rather than $400,000 over the period in question, the amount appeared to be $4,000 during Norris's time as administrator, or a little over $200 a year split among the typing pool.

The money, the commissioner's report concluded, had never been shared with Norris or any member of the scientific staff. The investigators found that Norris "had no connection with the alleged illegal practices." The chief medical examiner had, instead, "paid substantial amounts [out] of his own pocket for the expenses of his office."

Norris accepted the findings with dignity, but he was incensed. When he was asked to join in a tribute to Mayor La Guardia, he wrote back that he was afraid he just couldn't do that. He didn't know the mayor well enough to comment on his good qualities.

Then Dr. Norris went on another, too-rare vacation. He was tired, damn tired, of all of it.

Norris returned from his vacation in late August, having enjoyed a leisurely cruise to the tropical climate of South America. He was still curiously weary though, moving slowly at the office. He laughed about it a little. He was sixty-seven years old, after all. Maybe he was just getting too old for the job.

On the morning of September 11, he woke up acutely nauseated. His doctor thought he had brought back a case of dysentery from his travels, but Norris grew steadily weaker all day. He died in his bed at eight-thirty that night. The cause was given as heart failure, although many of his friends considered that he had, most probably, worked himself to death.

More than three hundred people attended his funeral at St. Thomas Episcopal Church, at Fifth Avenue and 53rd Street. Thirty uniformed policemen, including five on horseback, formed an honor guard around the entrance. His coffin lay at the front of the church, covered with ferns and banked with red roses, and as the choir sang "Onward Christian Soldiers," policemen carried it down the aisle, followed by his wife, Eugenie, his sister, his niece, and her husband. His daughter, vacationing in Europe at the time of his death, was still trying to get home.

The chairman of the state liquor authority was there, as were the assistant chief inspector of police, the commissioner of hospitals, the president of the Academy of Medicine, the director of the Bellevue laboratories, the dean of the NYU medical school, the chief medical examiner of Boston, and the head of the New York Medical Association. Harrison Martland was there. So was Thomas Gonzales, who had taken over as acting medical examiner. So were physicians, chemists, clerks, and stenographers from the medical examiner's offices. Alexander Gettler, city toxicologist, sat quietly in one of the front pews.

The New York papers listed every dignitary at the funeral. The list did not include Mayor La Guardia. But Norris, the constant gadfly, would undoubtedly have laughed about that.

And he would surely have been touched by the respect and affection shown by those who worked closely with him.

The staff took up a collection to have a portrait of him painted and hung in the main office. Everyone donated: stenographers and clerks, pathologists and chemists, his longtime chauffeur, and the cleaning woman. Gonzales organized a fund for a Charles Norris Fellowship in Forensic Medicine, to support promising students in the new NYU program. As Gonzales wrote to one contributor, no one was surprised by the generous response, "because of the great friendship and admiration of so many, like yourself, for Doctor Norris." Tributes came from around the world, across the country, but the most fervent came from those who'd worked alongside him.

A letter from the medical examiner on Staten Island was typical. It began on a stately note, praising Norris's skills as a pathologist and his pioneering work in making forensic medicine a respected science. And it closed on a personal one: "In sending my small contribution I am expressing my gratitude to the Chief for his friendship, for the many personal acts of assistance, for his extremely generous and whole-hearted support when most I needed it in my early days in the office, for his stimulating and encouraging words and cheery smile specially at moments when the difficulties of the office made all the world seem rather bleak."

But perhaps the best way to appreciate Charles Norris and what he had accomplished was to observe the New York City medical examiner's office at work. Norris's carefully built team of forensic detectives — with their hard-earned reputation for excellence, and their insistence on training and scientific procedure — would be well challenged in the days following his funeral.

They found much of it predictable — the auto accidents, the alcoholic collapses, the shootings and beatings, the familiar back-beat of life in the way it too often goes wrong. In the autumn following Norris's death, the department would work with police in investigating a butler who had stirred lead acetate into his mean-spirited employer's soup; a paintbrush salesman who slashed a friend's throat in a Broadway cafeteria because he suspected him of sleeping with his wife; a subway porter in Queens who stabbed a man who refused to tip; and a night watchman who killed a seventy-one-year-old baker for his payroll money. The deaths continued in that seemingly inevitable rhythm that Norris had known, fought, and sometimes simply mourned.

Still, there was one case, less than two weeks after his funeral, that would stand out from the steady patter of death — a killing made memorable by its chilly calculation, its sexually twisted motives, and by the fact that one of the suspects had an uncomfortably recognizable face, at least to Alexander Gettler.

The case began in mid-September, when a thirty-six-year-old Long Island housewife suddenly fell desperately sick, vomiting constantly, doubled over with abdominal pains. Her doctor, suspecting a gallbladder attack, sent Ada Appelgate to the hospital. She returned home after a week, still a little shaky on her feet, and went straight to her bed, still wretched enough that she refused food, drinking only milk, sometimes with a little egg and sugar mixed into it.

Two days later, on September 27, she woke up again violently ill, falling rapidly into unconsciousness. Her husband, Everett, called the doctor and the police, begging for someone to bring oxygen. When the doctor arrived, the police were still trying to coax breath from a dead woman. The doctor had been treating Ada for obesity for some time. She weighed almost 270 pounds — and he decided that her overtaxed heart must have finally failed. He wrote "coronary occlusion" on the death certificate and had the body sent to a funeral home.

That might have been that, except that the Appelgates shared their home with a rather notorious couple who had once been tried for arsenic murder: John and Mary Frances Creighton.

The Creightons had been living quietly since their acquittals some twelve years earlier. They'd sold their house in New Jersey and bought a small bungalow in the Long Island town of Baldwin. John had taken a job in the county engineer's office. Their children, Ruth, now fifteen, and Jack, twelve, attended the local schools.

During this time John had joined the American Legion. His friends in the lodge included Everett Appelgate, who was a local officer in the organization. Appelgate worked as an investigator in the Veterans'

Relief Bureau, and he and his wife and daughter lived with her parents. After the Appelgates quarreled with Ada's father, Creighton offered to let them live in the bungalow for a share of the costs. The home had only two bedrooms on its ground floor. The adults took those; Ruth and the Appelgates' daughter, Agnes, slept in the attic; and Jackie Creighton slept on a cot set out on the porch.

It was crowded, too cozy maybe, but "the Great Depression was with us," wrote the journalist Dorothy Kilgallen, who would cover the murder trial on Long Island, "and the idea of two families sharing so small a home was not likely to startle anyone."

None of the neighbors particularly liked Ada. She had a habit of criticizing people who annoyed her, which seemed to be almost everyone. But the two families seemed to get along just fine; no one knew of any trouble in the home on Bryant Place.

After her death, given the Creightons' history, the police asked Appelgate if they could order an autopsy on his wife. To their surprise, he refused. The district attorney called Appelgate to tell him that his office could compel an autopsy, but it would look better if the husband agreed.

After Appelgate reluctantly consented,

pathologists removed the dead woman's organs and sent them to Gettler's laboratory. He reported back that he'd found arsenic in every organ; he calculated that Ada must have received more than three times the lethal dose. After a few more days of investigation, on October 6, the Nassau County police charged Mary Frances Creighton — currently calling herself Fran — and Everett Appelgate with murder.

The reappearance of Mary Frances Creighton gave Gettler a jolt.

As Kilgallen pointed out in her account of the trial, he'd been a defense witness in one of her earlier arsenic murder trials. His own chemical analysis had helped clear her of the accusation that she'd murdered her mother-in-law.

The new investigation — to his very probable relief — found no evidence that he'd been wrong in that case. But it strongly suggested that she'd outwitted detection in the other charge, the murder of her brother. During interviews with a psychologist hired by the police department, Mary Frances confided that she had actually killed her teenage sibling; she'd wanted the insurance money. Her poison of choice at the time had been not the dilute Fowler's Solution (which the police had found) but the pesticide Rough on Rats, which she'd managed to throw away.

That arsenic-rich formula was also the poison that Gettler found in Ada Appelgate's body, right down to the other ingredients mixed into the rat bait. It followed the pattern that forensic scientists had observed even in the nineteenth century. Arsenic killers were often so successful with their first murder that they tended to believe they could get away with it again.

Creighton had not aged well in the years since the 1923 murder trials. Her dark Madonna looks were gone. She appeared older than her thirty-six years, squat and triple-chinned; in photographs, she had an oddly froglike look. Her alleged co-conspirator, Everett Appelgate, was exactly her age but looked much younger. He was trim, brown-haired, and blue-eyed, proud of his looks. When detectives asked him if his relationship with Fran Creighton could be a motive for murder, he hurriedly denied it. They were housemates and friends, he said, and that was all there was to it.

The police were only slightly off target, though. And the correct answer explained why a top-dog journalist like Kilgallen, of

Hearst's *New York Journal American,* would cover a seedy suburban murder case. And why she would title her account of the trial "Poison and Pedophilia."

Appelgate wasn't having an affair with Mary Frances Creighton. He was enjoying one with her rather beautiful fifteen-year-old daughter.

Q. You had intercourse with Ruth in the very bed where your wife lay?

A. Yes.

Q. What did your wife say to that?

A. She didn't know anything about the intercourse.

Q. You were nude?

A. Yes.

Q. Was your wife nude?

A. Yes.

Q. And Ruth slept nude?

A. She came in clothed.

Q. But she soon stripped.

A. Yes.

Q. So we have a picture of your wife and Ruth and you in this bed, nude?

A. Yes.

The trial began on January 13, 1936.

Appelgate testified that he'd wanted to marry Ruth Creighton. Although he denied that Ada had known about the affair, witnesses said differently.

Ruth testified that Appelgate had once asked her if she would like him better if he were single. She also recounted an incident in which she was riding home in the Appelgates' car. The couple was quarreling. When they got to the house, Ada slammed out of the car. Her husband came after her, knocking her to the ground. She got up, screaming at him, "If it was Ruth, you wouldn't have done that."

John Creighton was also called as a witness. He told of a Labor Day party when the Appelgates again quarreled and Everett slapped his wife in the face and shoved her down into a chair. She snapped at him, "If you ever do that again, I will tell something that will put you where you belong."

Creighton admitted to being puzzled at the time. Later Appelgate told him he wished he could put Ruth in an apartment "and keep her there and not have her around the house, and if she got in trouble, I could get a doctor to fix her up." He said, "What do you think of that?"

Creighton testified that he was dumbfounded, saying, "What do you mean by that, Appy? You wouldn't do anything to my daughter, would you?"

Appelgate, he said, had completely denied it: "No, sir. You know me. I would not harm a hair of her head."

John Creighton had believed his friend. It appeared now he'd been wrong, not to say stupid, about it.

According to Appelgate, John was the only innocent parent in the Creighton family. He testified that Mary Frances had known that Ruth was sleeping with him; she was even helping him keep track of Ruth's menstrual periods. She liked the idea of her daughter being married and out of the overcrowded house.

Appelgate admitted that he'd driven Mary Frances to a cut-rate drugstore to buy a packet of Rough on Rats and had given her the money for it. But he insisted that she had told him that she needed the poison to deal with some mice in the house. He had been shocked, he said, when his wife died. Mary Frances testified that he had taken her to the drugstore and given her twenty-five cents to get rat powder, then taken it from her and put it in his pocket.

About the night of the murder, she said: "Shortly after dinner that night, I went to the icebox and got the milk and poured it into a glass and he gave me or handed me a powder and told me to put it in the milk. Sort of a grayish white substance, a white paper."

Q. You knew the powder was arsenic?
A. Only his saying so.
Q. So when you put that eggnog on Ada's table and waited for her to drink it, you knew there was arsenic in it?
A. That's true.
Q. And you stood by and watched her die?
A. I didn't know she was dying.
Q. You didn't know she was dying?
A. Well — not exactly.

On January 30 Mary Frances Creighton and Everett Appelgate were convicted of first-degree murder and sentenced to die at Sing Sing. In May the New York Court of Appeals upheld the decision in both cases, noting that Creighton was "proved guilty beyond reasonable doubt" and that "as to Appelgate, the jury were justified in finding him guilty. His motive for disposing of her is apparent . . . his conduct speaks for himself."

The execution of the two killers was scheduled for July 16 at eleven o'clock at night. It was relatively quiet at the prison.

These weren't the kind of killers to draw an overflowing crowd. They hadn't aroused the sympathetic fascination that Ruth Snyder compelled almost a decade earlier. But the journalists following the case were there, sitting on those same hard wooden pews, watching convicted killers strapped into the harness of that same black chair.

Appelgate walked steadily to his seat, determinedly calm. As the guards fastened the straps, he said only, "Before I die, I say I am innocent of this crime." Mary Frances had to be wheeled into the room. She was so terrified that she couldn't walk. As they rolled her into the Death House, she was clutching a rosary. She had met with the prison chaplain that afternoon, who persuaded her that some additional faith in God might help. A longtime Protestant, she'd been baptized a Catholic at four o'clock that afternoon, agreeing that "it will make it easier for me to die."

She said nothing as she was settled into the chair. But just before the current went on, she threw the rosary beads to the floor.

The Creighton conviction must have been bittersweet for Gettler, who was no doubt tormented by the role he played in exonerating Creighton some twelve years before.

Yet while the first trial served as a plaguing reminder of science's fallibility, the second trial was testament to the great progress Gettler and his colleagues had made in earning forensic toxicology a place of respect in the courtroom. During Creighton's first trial for the death of her brother, defense attorneys had been able to mock the prosecution's scientific evidence. By the time of her second trial, defense attorneys were complaining that the city lab's reputation was too strong, and that Gettler was so well respected that jurors tended to accept whatever he said.

This dramatic shift in popular opinion was made possible by Norris and Gettler's unfaltering dedication to furthering the study of forensic toxicology. Norris and Gettler's often thankless work — the long nights in the laboratory, the endless fights with the mayor's office, the battles against the federal government and big business alike — had produced real results. Norris and Gettler had, indeed, changed the poison game.

The triumph of the Creighton trial — an act of justice made possible by scientific evidence — belonged to both men, and though Norris was not alive to celebrate the accomplishment, a picture of the two colleagues, taken about a year before the trial in their Bellevue laboratory, pays tribute to the work they did together. In that scene, now filed away in the city's archive, Norris perches on a stool, bent over a microscope that sits on a long table cluttered with glass beakers and notebooks. Gettler leans over his shoulder, face intent. One can almost hear his voice, soft yet serious in explanation. The photograph is black and white, of course, but we can well imagine that lights above their heads glowed with gold incandescence and the Bunsen burner flames, on the lab bench behind them, shimmered a pale unearthly blue. Perhaps it was late in the evening — as it often was when they conducted their tests — and darkness was gathering outside amber-lit windows. It would have been quiet in the lab, peacefully so, but they would have known that out in the shadows, another poisoner was waiting in the dark, planning his next move.

# EPILOGUE:
# THE SUREST POISON

Tobacco, coffee, alcohol, hashish, prussic acid, strychnine, are weak dilutions: the surest poison is time.
> — RALPH WALDO EMERSON,
> "Old Age," *Atlantic Monthly,*
> January 1862

At the time of Norris's death, Thomas Gonzales and two other medical examiners in the Manhattan office — Morgan Vance and Milt Helpern — were working on a comprehensive textbook on forensic science. *Legal Medicine and Toxicology* was published two years later and dedicated to Norris. When the authors published a second edition in 1954, they updated the procedures and poisons, but the dedication remained as ever: "To the memory of Charles Norris, First Chief Medical Examiner of The City of New York."

Alexander Gettler remained New York City's chief toxicologist until January 1, 1959, retiring at the age of seventy-five. The mandatory retirement age was seventy, but the city approved a special dispensation in his case. On the day he left office, he estimated that he'd analyzed more than 100,000 bodies.

He'd also published a library's worth of papers — work on ethyl and methyl alcohol, cyanide, carbon monoxide, fluoride, chloroform, benzene, thallium, the micro-isolation of volatile toxic substances from tissues, investigations of the Reinsch test, and occasionally casework that had nothing to do with a poison. He also helped train that new generation of forensic toxicologists — that special club known as the Gettler Boys — who would go on to head forensic laboratories from Long Island to Puerto Rico.

One of Gettler's former students, Abraham Freireich, who worked on the alcohol intoxication studies and was a founding member of the Academy of Forensic Sciences' toxicology division, echoed the comments of many when he wrote, "If any one person deserves the appellation 'father of toxicology and forensic chemistry in the United States,' it is Dr. Gettler."

Henry Freimuth, who worked with Gettler on his studies of carbon monoxide poisoning and later became head toxicologist at the chief medical examiner's office in Baltimore, Maryland, pointed out that all of Gettler's tests were done with what toxicologists now call "wet" chemistry, relying on test tubes and Bunsen burners, beakers and body parts. To check and recheck his results on alcohol content in the brain, for instance, Gettler sometimes needed half a pound of tissue, compared to the bare smear of material used in the "dry" chemistry enabled by newer machines.

The work was so often grisly that Gettler created a test of laboratory applicants' fortitude. He kept a white enameled can of disintegrating brain tissue in the refrigerator. Potential toxicologists would be asked to use it in a demonstration of distillation, first by grinding the decaying brain tissue into a slurry of grayish slime. As it oozed over the applicants' gloves, the queasy among them bolted from the laboratory. "If they did not, they then passed the first step of their evaluation," wrote Irving Sunshine, who passed the test, studied under Gettler, and went on to become one of the country's leading forensic toxicologists, teaching at Cleveland's Case Western University while serving as chief toxicologist for Ohio's

Cuyahoga County.

Sunshine helped pioneer the profession's shift from wet chemistry to dry, using sensitive instruments such as the gas chromatograph and mass spectrometer, which could process trace samples. He believed this shift was so important that he often worked directly with equipment manufacturers and tested prototype machines in his laboratory. The machines, Sunshine said, were needed in an era when poisonous new compounds were being developed at a rate far eclipsing that of the early twentieth century.

But consider, he added, the even greater challenge to Alexander Gettler, at a time when everything depended on the scientist's intuition and inventiveness — and absolute understanding of chemical reactions. Gettler had once sat up all night building a tiny apparatus to collect drips of chemical solution from an infant's brain — to show that a nurse, overenthusiastically applying medicine for a lice infection, had poisoned the baby. Gettler and his crew of young chemists "laid the foundation on which today's relatively esoteric technology is based," Sunshine said. "They could function with a test tube and a beaker. Where would today's toxicologist be if the electricity shuts down?"

Unlike his famous chief, Charles Norris,

who frequently used his position as a public platform, Gettler was an essentially private man in a visible job. He turned down a proposal for a television series based on his work because his wife hated the idea. His students recalled his eccentricities with affection — the way he'd sneak away every day to call his bookie, his addiction to horse racing, his passionate love of the Yankees and card games. They remembered the way he'd stand, shirtsleeves rolled up and cigar tucked in a corner of his mouth, and survey a tray filled with beakers containing treated liver extracts, then identify the poison. "Few ever had the privilege of watching 'the old man' do the classical color spot tests [such as those used in search of the blue of cyanide] on these residues," Sunshine wrote. "However, everyone marveled at how well he identified the offending agents."

But when interviewed about his work, Gettler retreated into propriety like a turtle into a shell. He was so careful about the information he shared that sometimes he gave out no information at all. He had the personality of a clerk, wrote one journalist. He would be more famous, said another, if he weren't so pedantic. In a 1955 profile, "The Man Who Reads Corpses," published in *Harper's,* the writer described the toxicologist as "a crusty, precise man of seventy, barely saved from an air of primness by an ever-present cigar."

Several years after he retired, Gettler suffered a stroke. It slowed him down; he took to walking with a cane. He and his wife, Alice, moved from Brooklyn to Yonkers, to be closer to their son, Joseph, a chemistry professor at Columbia University, and his family. He died on August 4, 1968, and was buried in the Gate of Heaven Cemetery in Hawthorne. "His interest in his former students and assistants never abated," Abe Freireich wrote. "On visiting him just a short time before his death, the entire afternoon was spent in bringing him up to date on the whereabouts and activities of his former disciples. His influence lives on in most of the major toxicology laboratories in the country."

Gettler's own assessment was typically more modest. In a fleeting moment of openness, he admitted to the *Harper's* correspondent that for all his obsession with detail, the carefully repeated experiments, the data bank of chemical information that he'd built up over the years, the results still weighed on him. His chemistry had helped the innocent escape murder charges — Charles Webb, Frank Travia, Frederick

Gross. But it had also helped convict and send others — Ruth Snyder and Judd Gray, Tony Marino and the Mike Malloy conspirators, Mary Frances Creighton and Everett Appelgate — to the electric chair.

His son, Joseph, a theoretical chemist, had once announced that he'd decided early on against forensic toxicology: he could never have so many lives and deaths on his conscience. His father understood him. Because sometimes the dead did walk in Alexander Gettler's sleep, sometimes they rattled in the black chair of Sing Sing, and always, as he admitted in that last vulnerable interview, "I keep asking myself, have I done everything right?"

# AUTHOR'S NOTE

When I went to college, I dreamed of becoming a chemist (which my children assure me reveals the true geekiness at the core of my personality). I changed my mind on the day that I set my hair on fire — think long, dangling 1970s braids, think Bunsen burner. "Do you smell smoke?" the graduate student running the classroom laboratory inquired. Or it might have been the day that I smoked out the entire room due to a certain incident involving toxic fumes that I prefer to forget.

A chemistry lab is a dangerous place for an absentminded daydreamer of a student — in other words, me. But put a focused and meticulous scientist there instead and he or she can illuminate the intricate, internal machinery of anything from a crystal of sugar to the labyrinthine structure of strychnine. I still remember that dazzle of realization from my classes. It's probably one of the reasons I occasionally, wistfully, describe myself as a lapsed chemist, although we're talking about a lapse of decades.

Even such a brief foray into chemistry teaches that anything, in a large enough amount, can kill. Life-giving water itself is lethal if you gulp down too many gallons. As toxicologists say, the dose makes the poison. But poison by water doesn't unnerve us. The real scare comes from those elements and compounds whose toxicity is measured in drips and drops. Luckily for us, and other life on Earth, such materials are rare. But somehow we've managed to find or create many of them. We use them pragmatically, and for good — our medicine relies on countless toxic compounds — and in deliberate evil.

There exists a kind of murder mystery pleasure to the subject of poisons; crime novelists, especially in the early twentieth century, have written them into countless tales of deathly intrigue. I've always admired the stylish writing of those vintage novels, which is a nice way of saying that I've read and enjoyed numerous stories involving murder by arsenic and cyanide. That hasn't affected the fact that, in reality, I find poison killings among the most disturbing of all homicides.

I see poisoners — so calculating, so cold-blooded — as most like the villains of our horror stories. They're closer to that lurking monster in the closet than some drug-impaired crazy with a gun. I don't mean to dismiss the latter — both can achieve the same awful results. But the scarier killer is the one who thoughtfully plans his murder ahead, tricks a friend, wife, lover into swallowing something that will dissolve tissue, blister skin, twist the muscles with convulsions, *knows* all that will happen and does it anyway.

The fact of homicidal poisoning shows us at our amoral worst. The fact that most of us regard it with revulsion, work so hard to detect and punish it, defies that conclusion. It reminds us that human decency largely prevails. Both those sides of our nature are revealed in the history of poisons. I believe the quest for moral balance holds center in this story and that it outshines, in the end, even the creepy charm of the poisoners among us. But I've learned, along the way, that we never quite leave behind the monster in the closet. There are mornings, lit by the cold winter light, when I start talking about a poison in my book, revealing my own dangerous expertise, and as I do, I watch

my husband quietly, not really thinking
about it, slide his cup out of my reach.

Deborah Blum
Madison, Wisconsin
May 2009

# GRATITUDES

It's been a privilege to write about Charles Norris and Alexander Gettler. Mostly forgotten by our generation, they were revolutionaries who worked in civil service, and that as we all know, is something to be celebrated. I am grateful for the opportunity to tell their story, and I am grateful for — and blessed in — all the people who helped me to do so:

My always amazing agent, Suzanne Gluck, who said to me, "Why don't you write that poison book you've always wanted to do?" and then made sure that I could.

My always wonderful editor, Ann Godoff, who took a chance on my initial rather dreamy idea, patiently helped me pull all the disparate elements together, and made it a much better (and smarter) book.

The rest of the great staff at Penguin Press, with special thanks to Lindsay Whalen, Beena Kamlani, Caroline Garner, and Janet Biehl, for all their terrific help.

The Alfred P. Sloan Foundation and, in particular, vice president for programs Doron Weber — for believing that the chemistry woven through this book mattered and for giving me a grant that allowed me to do the necessary research.

The Graduate School of the University of Wisconsin, Madison, which provided summer money so that I could concentrate on just writing, and especially Ernesto Livorni, who argued my case but later confided that the desperate quality of my application — "I have a deadline, help, help!" — provided him with real entertainment.

My terrific graduate researcher, Kajsa Dalrymple, who spent hours studying obscure poisons and poisoners, finding scientific journals of the 1920s and 1930s, contacting archivists and toxicologists around the country, digging through archives, and reading microfiche of long-gone New York newspapers — and supported my idea of drinking our way through the catalog of Prohibition-era cocktails. We didn't get very far, but I do highly recommend the Bee's Knees.

The incredibly generous family of Alexander O. Gettler: daughter-in-law Mary Gettler, grandson Paul Gettler, granddaughter Dorothy Atzl, and great-granddaughter, Vicky Atzl. They not only took time out from their busy schedules to meet with me, but they hunted up family documents and memorabilia. Dorothy and Vicky shared with me the really incredible research from an honors presentation that Vicky had done on her great-grandfather, which included letters, published papers, and even videotapes. I can't say thank you enough.

The staff at the New York City Municipal Archive, who unearthed stacks of boxes containing the correspondence from Charles Norris's term as city medical examiner; archivist Nancy Miller from the University of Pennsylvania, who collected background information on early American toxicology for me, above and beyond; Jennifer Comins, of the Columbia University Archives, who tracked down the alumni information on Norris and Gettler; Stephen Bohlen, of the communications office at Bellevue Hospital, who not only gave me a tour of the hospital's past but let me rummage through the history files; the librarians at the New York Public Library and the New York Historical Society, who helped me gather resources on jazz-age New York.

A special note of gratitude to Mary Hitchcock, medical history librarian at the University of Wisconsin's Ebling Health Sciences Library, who can find anything and who saved my tail when I was seeking information on thallium in the 1930s.

Forensic toxicologist extraordinaire John Trestrail III, who allowed me to pester him with all kinds of questions — and answered them all with supporting documentation.

Two renowned chemists, Bassam Shakashiri, of the University of Wisconsin, and Harry Gray, of the California Institute of Technology, who helped me figure out carbon monoxide poisoning at the molecular level, so that I could understand why Alexander Gettler's color results worked the way they did. Yes, I am that obsessive.

Three of the best friends ever, who read the manuscript for me: Robin Marantz Henig, who helped me clarify many of the early chapters; Kim Fowler, who rescued it from typos and tense problems; and Denise Allen, who cheered me on while providing me with an outstanding selection of early-twentieth-century crime fiction.

And almost last — but never least — my sons, Marcus and Lucas Haugen, whose imitations of me as a parent — "Go away. I'm working on my book" — are unfortunately accurate at least some of the time.

They make me laugh, and despite their sarcasm, they make me happy. As does my husband, Peter. He bravely read the manuscript and improved it in countless ways. I promise publicly — his coffee is safe from me forever.

# A GUIDE TO THE HANDBOOK

We are like dwarfs sitting on the shoulders of giants. We see more, and things that are more distant, than they did, not because our sight is superior or because we are taller than they, but because they raise us up, and by their great stature add to ours.

— JOHN OF SALISBURY,
*Metalogicon,* 1159

If I have seen farther, it is by standing on the shoulders of giants.

— SIR ISAAC NEWTON,
letter to Robert Hooke,
February 15, 1676

As my book is about Charles Norris, Alexander Gettler, and the toxicology of the early twentieth century, the focus is on their work and their place in history. But, many other scientists contributed to the field, from those who first attempted to catch poisoners in earlier centuries, to those doing work today. Dedicated researchers working in numerous countries built the field of forensic toxicology, advance by advance. Today's toxicologists stand on the work of Gettler, Norris, and their contemporaries, just as they themselves did on previous generations. On the history and scope of the work, the volumes that I found most useful include:

Autenrieth, Wilhelm, and W. H. Warren. *Laboratory Manual for the Detection of Poisons and Powerful Drugs* (London: J & A Churchill, 1928).

Bamford, Frank. *Poisons: Their Isolation and Identification* (London: J & A Churchill, 1947).

Boos, William F. *The Poison Trail* (Boston: Hale, Cushman & Flint, 1939).

Christison, Robert. *A Treatise on Poisons* (Philadelphia: Ed. Barrington and Geo. D. Haswell, Philadelphia, 1845).

Emsley, John. *The Elements of Murder: A History of Poison* (New York: Oxford University Press, 2006).

Essig, Mark R. *Science and Sensation: Poison Murder and Forensic Science in Nineteenth Century America* (Ph.D. diss.,

Cornell University, 2000).

Gerber Samuel, ed. *Chemistry and Crime* (Washington, D.C.: American Chemical Society, 1983).

Gerber, Samuel, and Richard Saferstein, eds. *More Chemistry and Crime* (Washington, D.C.: American Chemical Society, 1997).

Glaister, John. *The Power of Poison* (New York: William Morrow & Co., 1954).

Gonzales, Thomas, et al. *Legal Medicine: Pathology and Toxicology* (New York: Appleton-Century-Crofts, 1954).

Gonzales, Thomas, Morton Vance, and Milton Helpern. *Legal Medicine and Toxicology.* (New York Appleton-Century Co., 1937).

Grant, Julius. *Science for the Prosecution* (London: Chapman & Hall, 1941).

Lucas, A. *Forensic Chemistry and Scientific Criminal Investigation* (London: Edward Arnold & Co., 1921).

Magath, Thomas B., ed. *The Medicolegal Necropsy: A Symposium Held at the Twelfth Annual Convention of the American Society of Clinical Pathologists at Milwaukee, Wisconsin, June 9, 1933* (Baltimore: Williams & Wilkens Co., 1934).

Marten, Edward, and Beverly Leonidas

Clarke. *The Doctor Looks at Murder* (New York: Blue Ribbon Books, 1940).

McLaughlin, Terence. *The Coward's Weapon* (London: Robert Hale, 1980).

Mitchell, C. Ainsworth. *Science and the Criminal* (Boston: Little, Brown & Co., 1911).

Peterson, Frederick, Walter S. Haines, and Ralph Webster, eds. *Legal Medicine and Toxicology* (Philadelphia: W. B. Saunders Co., 1923).

Smith, John Gordon. *The Principles of Forensic Medicine* (London: Thomas & George Underwood, 1821).

Smith, Sydney. *Forensic Medicine* (London: J & A Churchill, 1940).

Sunshine, Irving, ed. *Was It a Poisoning? Forensic Toxicologists Searching for Answers* (New York: American Academy of Forensic Scientists/Society of Forensic Toxicologists, 1998).

Thompson, C. J. S. *Poison Mysteries in History, Romance and Crime* (Philadelphia: J. B. Lippincott Co., 1923).

Thorwald, Jürgen. *The Century of the Detective* (New York: Harcourt, Brace & World, 1965).

———. *Dead Men Tell Tales* (London: Thames & Hudson, 1966).

Ullyett, Kenneth. *Crime Out of Hand* (London: Michael Joseph, 1963).

Von Oettingen, W. F. *Poisoning* (London: Wm. Heinemann, 1952).

Witthaus, Rudolph, and Tracy Becker. *Medical Jurisprudence, Forensic Medicine and Toxicology,* Vol. 4. (New York: William Wood & Co., 1896).

These books provided the background for the overview of forensic toxicology contained in my prologue and you will also find them referenced in the chapter notes pertaining to the history of different poisons, as well as other materials specific to individual cases. Collectively, they stand as a reminder that even such innovative scientists as Charles Norris and Alexander Gettler "stand on the shoulders of giants" and thrive in the company of friends.

# NOTES

**1. Chloroform**

**when ice storms had glassed over . . . :**
"Blanket of Ice Covers the City," *New York Times,* February 3, 1915, p. 5.

**Typhoid Mary had come sneaking back . . . :** "Caught at Last," *New York Sun,* March 31, 1915, p. 6; "Typhoid Mary Reappears," *New York Tribune,* March 29, 1915, p. 8.

**Instead, Patrick Riordan . . . :** "Wallstein Attacks Coroner Riordan," *New York Times,* January 10, 1915, p. 20; "Shonts asks for Coroner's Removal," *New York Times,* January 28, 1915, p. 8; "Riordan Drunk, Murphy Declares: Assistant District Attorney Tells of His Conduct at Accident Inquest," *New York Times,* April 7, 1915, p. 6.

**Frederic Mors was a small man . . . :** The story of Frederic Mors appears on

Wikipedia, where he is cited as a serial killer: http://en.wikipedia.org/wiki/ Frederick_Mors. In a catalog of serial killers on the true crime website CrimeZZZ .net, he can be found under the name Carl Menarik: http://www.crimezzz.net/ serialkillers/M/MENARIK_carl.php.

**He'd found a job as an orderly . . . :** The "Squad Room" blog names the German Odd Fellows home as the "the scene of the first mass murder by a serial killer to be investigated by the NYPD": http:// brooklynnorth.blogspot.com/2002_03_01 _archive.html. The Odd Fellows home, by all accounts, was not a very nice place, even aside from providing a base for a serial killer. Newspaper accounts report that it took state money to provide vocational training for orphans and then, rather than training them, put them to work doing menial chores. An investigation by New York City's commissioner of charities concluded that it was representative of foundling homes in which "peonage" and "child labor" were part of the basic operation.

**"It was really a kind-hearted thing . . .":** Mors is routinely written up as a serial killer, despite the failure of the investigating officials even to send him to trial. Most of my research into his story comes from newspaper accounts, including these from *New York Times:* "Killed 8 In Home He Tells Perkins," February 3, 1915, p. 9; "Indorse Queer Tale of Killing The Aged," February 6, 1915, p. 1; "May Indict Three For Deaths in Home," February 7, 1915, p. 1; "Chloroform Burns Point to Murders," February 8, 1915, p. 1; "Girl Saw Mors in Death Chamber," February 9, 1915, p. 1; "Deaths Continued After Mors Denial," February 10, 1915, p.1; "Mors Killed As Act of Kindness, He Says," February 12, 1915, p. 6; "Mors May Go Free Despite 8 Deaths," February 11, 1915, p. 18; "May Not Try Mors on Murder Charge," February 13, 1915, p. 10; "Bangert Confronts His Poison Accuser," February 15, 1915, p. 5; "Mors Escapes From Asylum," May 12, 1916, p. 11.

**There wasn't a cop in the room . . . :** The history of chloroform is the subject of a fascinating book by Linda Stratmann, *Chloroform: The Quest for Oblivion* (Phoenix Mill, Gloustershire: Sutton, 2003). See also Witthaus and Becker, *Medical Jurisprudence,* pp. 850–54; Peterson, Haines, and Webster, *Legal Medicine,* pp. 639–49; Gonzales, Vance, and Helpern, *Legal Medicine and Toxicology,* pp. 742–45; Gonzales et al., *Pathology and Toxicology,* pp. 795–96.

**It was the case of Texas multimillionaire William Rice . . . :** The website of Houston's Rice University notes that "William Rice [was] murdered" on September 23, 1900, and that Albert Patrick was jailed the following year. It does not mention his later release. On the mysterious nature of Rice's death, as well as the conflicting medical testimony, see the true crime Web site "The Malfactor's Register," http://markgribben.com/?page_id=61; Marguerite Johnston, *Houston: The Unknown City* (College Station: Texas A&M University Press, 1991), pp. 117–23; and the online legal encyclopedia, *Law Library: American Law and Legal Information: Great American Trials,* vol. 1, http://law.jrank.org/pages/2737/Albert-Patrick-Trial-1902.html. I also reviewed the *New York Times* coverage: "Cause of Death: Patrick's Counsel Try to Prove It Was Due to Heart Disease," February 4, 1902, p. 16; "Jones Tells How He Murdered Rice," February 21, 1902, p. 2; "Patrick Defense Opens: Counsel Will Try to Show That Rice Was Not Murdered," March 7, 1902, p. 7; "Dr.

Lee at Patrick Trial," March 11, 1902, p. 7; "Tests in Patrick Trial," March 13, 1902, p. 2; "Grover Cleveland Asks Clemency for Patrick," December 30, 1905, p. 4; "New Patrick Evidence for Last Appeal," January 14, 1906, p. 14; "Patrick Tells Why He Expects Pardon," December 19, 1910, p. 1; and "Dr. Flint Believes Patrick Innocent," December 20, 1910.

**Like all other buildings in New York, Bellevue and Allied Hospitals . . . :** See "Bellevue Hospital's Story," *New York Times,* April 18, 1926, p. XX18; "How the Bellevue Capitals Were Saved," *NYU Physician* (Fall 1990), pp. 47–48; Page Cooper, *The Bellevue Story* (New York: Thomas Y. Crowell Co., 1948), pp. 113–225; Sandra Opdyke, *No One Was Turned Away: The Role of Public Hospitals in New York City Since 1900* (New York: Oxford University Press, 1999); Bellevue Hospital Milestones, unpublished list, courtesy Bellevue Public Relations Office.

**The hospital's famed psychopathic ward . . . :** "Reception Hospitals, Psychopathic Wards and Psychopathic Hospitals," read at the meeting of the American Medico-Psychological Association, Washington, D.C., May 7, 1907, is a model of compassion and innovative thinking.

**That same January the city government had released a report . . . :** On Wallstein's report on the coroner system, see "Oust Coroners, Says Wallstein," *New York Times,* January 4, 1915, p. 1; and "Coroners' System Sheer Waste of Public Money," *New York Times,* January 10, 1915, p. 44. The dismal state of coroner operations in New York, before Charles Norris, and elsewhere was reviewed in "The Coroner and the Medical Examiner," *Bulletin of the National Research Council,* July 1928, no. 64; Luke May, *Crime's Nemesis* (New York: Macmillan: 1916), pp. 107–108; Julie Johnson, "Coroners, Corruption and the Politics of Death: Forensic Pathology in the United States," in Michael Clark and Catherine Crawford, eds., *Legal Medicine in History* (New York: Cambridge University Press, 1994), pp. 268–89.

**Yet the scientific journals supported . . . :** On chloroform knowledge at the time of the Mors case, see Witthaus and Becker, *Medical Jurisprudence,* pp. 850–54; Peterson, Haines, and Webster, *Legal Medicine;* Lucas, *Forensic Chemistry.*

## 2. Wood Alcohol

**As he liked to boast . . . :** The official biography of Mayor John F. "Red Mike" Hylan can be found on New York City's website: www.nyc.gov/html/nyc100/html/classroom/hist_info/mayors.html#hylan. He is also profiled in the online encyclopedia, NationMaster.com: www.nationmaster.com/encyclopedia/John-F.-Hylan and in "Sketches of American Mayors," *National Municipal Review,* 15, no. 3, (pp. 158–65).

**The tireless Leonard Wallstein . . . :** The political fight over the medical examiner's office was followed closely by the *New York Times:* "Civil Service Board Backs Hylan Move," January 14, 1918, p. 12; "Try to Stop Riordan's Pay," January 27, 1918, p. 14; "Move for Riordan by Civil Service," January 28, 1918, p. 5; "Civil Service Board Again Aids Riordan," January 29, 1918, p. 11; "Norris Succeeds Riordan," February 1, 1918, p. 10.

**"famed, sardonic, goat-bearded . . .":** *Time,* September 23, 1935 p. 27.

**Everyone knew that Norris didn't have to work . . . :** For Charles Norris biographic information, see "Resolutions Passed by the Faculty of Medicine of Columbia University on the Death of Dr.

Charles Norris," filed October 25, 1935, Columbia University archive; unpublished historical summary of Charles Norris's family history and life, including a list of scientific publications from the files of the medical examiner's office for 1918, New York City Municipal Archive; Frank J. Jirka, "A Great Scientific Detective," *American Doctors of Destiny* (Chicago: Normandie House, 1940), pp. 216–29; William G. Eckert, "Charles Norris (1868–1935) and Thomas A. Gonzales (1878–1956): New York's Forensic Pioneers," *American Journal of Forensic Medicine and Pathology* 8, no. 4 (1987), pp. 350–53.

**"A much neglected field of medical endeavor . . ."**: Draft editorial written for the *Journal of Forensic Medicine,* 1918, city examiner's file, New York City Municipal Archive.

**"We call this the Country Club"**: Milton Helpern and Bernard Knight, *Autopsy: The Memoirs of Milton Helpern, the World's Greatest Medical Detective* (New York: St. Martin's Press, 1977), p. 47.

**Norris had saved, with some enjoyment, the old coroner's . . . :** Riordan's inventory of possessions, January 8, 1918, medical examiner's files, New York City

Municipal Archive.

**Norris at least had a new home . . . :**
On Norris organizing the department, see
S. K. Niyogi, "Historic Development of
Forensic Toxicology in America up to
1978," *American Journal of Forensic Medicine and Pathology* 1, no. 3 (September
1980), pp. 249–64; W. G. Eckert, "Medicolegal Investigation in New York City:
History and Activities, 1918–1978," *American Journal of Forensic Medicine and Pathology* 4, no. 1 (March 1983), pp. 33–54.

**"the place for the laboratory force . . .":**
Charles Norris to John F. Hylan, December 18, 1918, medical examiner's file,
New York Municipal Archive.

**"useless timber":** Ibid.

**"This work, which I may term 'organization' . . .":** Ibid.

**"I wish to call to your attention . . .":**
Charles Norris to Richard Enright, police
commissioner, April 4, 1918, police department, New York City Municipal Archive.

**He wrote to the Bronx district attorney . . . :** Charles Norris to Seymour
Mork, assistant district attorney, Borough
of the Bronx, April 17, 1918, New York
City Municipal Archives.

**He wrote to hospitals . . . :** Charles Norris to George D. O'Hanlon, general medical superintendent, Bellevue and Allied Hospitals, April 16, 1918, New York City Municipal Archives.

**"Your peremptory order . . ."**; Superintendent of Methodist Episcopal Hospital to Charles Norris, June 7, 1918, New York City Municipal Archive.

**He was even tougher, though . . .** : Norris to Deputy Police Commissioner Lahey, April 19, 1918, New York City Municipal Archive.

**"Did you make any efforts . . ."**: Norris to Dr. George Teng, medical examiner's office, Brooklyn, June 10, 1918, New York City Municipal Archive.

**He chastised personnel . . .** : Norris to Dr. John Reigelman, medical examiner's office, Bronx, April 5, 1918, New York City Municipal Archive.

**Born in 1883, the son of a Hungarian . . .** : Alexander Gettler biographic information is from: Joseph Gettler, unpublished, handwritten tribute, and personal interviews, courtesy of the Gettler family; A. W. Freireich, "In Memoriam: Alexander O. Gettler, 1883–1968," *Journal of Forensic Sciences* 14, no. 3 (July 1969), pp. vii–xi; Henry C. Freimuth, "Alexander O. Gettler (1883–1968): A Reflection," *American Journal of Forensic Medicine and Pathology* 4, no. 4 (December 1983); The Toxicologist: A Modern Detective, November 25, 1933, p. 22; Sunshine, *Was It a Poisoning?;* Edward D. Radin, "The Professor Looks at Murder," in *12 Against Crime* (New York: G.P. Putnam's Sons, 1950); "The Chemistry of Crime," *Science Illustrated* 2, no. 5 (May 1947), pp. 44–47; Eugene Pawley, "Cause of Death: Ask Gettler," *American Mercury,* September 1954, pp. 62–66; "Test-tube Sleuth," *Time,* May 15, 1933; "The Man Who Reads Corpses," *Harper's Magazine,* February 1955, pp. 62–67.

**It would be a challenge . . . . :** Alexander O. Gettler, *The Historical Development of Toxicology,* presentation to the annual meeting of the American Academy of Forensic Sciences, Chicago, February 26–28, 1953.

**"Wood alcohol — technically known as methyl . . .":** Wood alcohol's chemical makeup is detailed at Medline Plus, www.nlm.nih.gov/medlineplus/ency/article/002827.htm. For alcohol history, see http://science.jrank.org/pages/186/Alcohol-History.html. A historical review more contemporary to my story is "Wood

Alcohol's Trail: Many Deaths Before Prohibition Throw Light on Methods Needed to Combat Evil," *New York Times,* January 15, 1922, p. 86.

**By the end of the nineteenth century . . . :** Information on the production and denaturing formulas in the early twentieth century can be found in Rufus Herrick, *Denatured or Industrial Alcohol* (New York: J. Wiley and Sons, 1907); H. W. Wiley, *Industrial Alcohol: Sources and Manufacture* (Washington, D.C.: U.S. Department of Agriculture, 1911).

**"The prohibition by our government . . .":** A. O. Gettler and A. V. St. George, "Wood Alcohol Poisoning," *Journal of the American Medical Association,* January 19, 1918, pp. 145–49. The uniquely poisonous metabolism of wood alcohol is discussed in this article and in John M. Robinson, "Blindness for Industrial Use of a .4 Per Cent Admixture of Wood Alcohol," *Journal of the American Medical Association,* January 19, 1918, pp. 148–49, and Charles Baskerville, "Wood Alcohol: Cooperative Caution," *Journal of Industrial and Engineering Chemistry,* January 1920, pp. 81–83.

**Poison was already in the air . . . :** International Film Service, "Mustard Gas

Warfare," *New York Times,* July 7, 1918, p. 52; "Vast U. S. Poison Plant Was Working at Full Blast for 1919 Campaign," *New York Times,* December 8, 1918, p. 45.

**On the home front . . . :** See "The Influenza Pandemic of 1918," http://virus.stanford.edu/uda/; "The Great Pandemic: State by State," www.pandemicflu.gov/general/greatpandemic2.html; "The Deadly Virus," www.archives.gov/exhibits/influenza-epidemic/records-list.html. On Bellevue's role in the influenza fight, see Sandra Opdycke, *No One Was Turned Away: The Role of Public Hospitals in New York City Since 1900* (New York: Oxford University Press, 1999); Page Cooper, *The Bellevue Story* (New York: T.Y. Crowell, 1948); and correspondence by Charles Norris.

**"Should any of our men . . .":** Norris to Major General Crowder, provost marshal general, Washington, D.C., September 6, 1918, medical examiner's files, New York City Municipal Archive.

**"During the years 1918 and 1919 . . .":** Alexander O. Gettler, "Critical Study of Methods for the Detection of Methyl Alcohol," *Journal of Biological Chemistry* 42, no. 2 (1920), pp. 311–28.

**"My attention has been called . . .":** Hylan to Norris, December 19, 1918, medical examiner's files, New York City Municipal Archive.

**"We have found . . .":** Norris to S. F. Wynne, Department of Health, medical examiner's files, New York City Municipal Archive.

**In December there had been forty-two . . . :** "Poison Drink Killed 51 Here; Blinded 100," *New York Times,* December 27, 1919, p. 3.

**As the month wound down . . .":** Ibid.

## 3. Cyanides

**Cocktail parties sparkled defiantly . . . :** For a good overview of Prohibition culture in New York City, see Michael A. Lerner, *Dry Manhattan* (Cambridge, Mass.: Harvard University Press, 2007).

**As soon as legal drinking ended . . . :** "Will Try to Indict for Poison Alcohol," *New York Times,* January 6, 1920, p. 4; "Four More Deaths from Wood Alcohol," *New York Times,* January 12, 1920, p. 10.

**"The speakeasies are . . .":** Stephen Graham, *New York Nights* (New York: George H. Doran Co., 1927), pp. 60–68.

**"Prohibition is a joke . . .":** "Prohibition a Joke, Dale Says on Bench," *New York Times,* August 12, 1920, p. 10.

**But for the new speakeasy devotees . . . :** Graham, *New York Nights.*

**They created a new generation of cock-tails . . . :** Recipes for 1920s cocktails can be found *in The Savoy Cocktail Book* (London: Constable and Co., 1930, re-printed London: Pavilion Books, 1999), among many other sources.

**a cloudy cocktail called Smoke . . . :** "Norris Explains Why the Death Rate Mounts," *New York World,* November 21, 1920, p. 3.

**As demands for chemical analysis in-tensified . . . :** Norris to John F. Hylan, June 12, 1922, medical examiner's files, New York City Municipal Archive.

**The Hotel Margaret glittered . . . :** Federal Writers Project, *The WPA Guide to New York City* (1939).

**"Mr. and Mrs. Jackson met their deaths . . .":** "Autopsy Deepens Jackson Mystery," *New York Times,* April 28, 1932, p. 36.

**Cyanides possess a uniquely long . . . :** On cyanides' history, chemical composi-tion, and uses, see Witthaus and Becker, *Medical Jurisprudence,* pp. 4: 602–40; Thompson, *Poison Mysteries,* pp. 143–76; Alexander O. Gettler and A. V. St. George, "Cyanide Poisoning," *American Journal of*

Clinical Pathology 4, no. 9 (September 1934) pp. 429–37.

**"The symptoms of acute poisoning . . .":** Gettler and St. George, "Cyanide Poisoning," p. 430.

**In the late 1890s one daring physician . . . :** Witthaus and Becker, Medical Jurisprudence, pp. 4: 610–12. The descriptions of internal damage and autopsy findings come from this source as well as Gettler and St. George, "Cyanide Poisoning"; Peterson, Haines, and Webster, Legal Medicine, pp. 674–82, and Gonzales et al., Pathology and Toxicology, pp. 802–804.

**In the four years since Gettler had become . . . :** Gettler and St. George, "Cyanide Poisoning," p. 433.

**So he set about doing the finer chemical tests . . . :** Gettler and St. George, "Cyanide Poisoning," pp. 435–37; Witthaus and Becker, Medical Jurisprudence, pp. 4: 610–12; Peterson, Haines, and Webster, Legal Medicine, pp. 680–82; Gonzales et al., Legal Medicine, pp. 1050–52.

**One of the most famous cyanide-by-mail murder cases . . . :** The story of the Molineux murders is beautifully told in Harold Schecter, The Devil's Gentleman: Privilege, Poison and the Trial That Ushered in the Twentieth Century (New York: Ballantine Books, 2007), and is recounted in numerous law and true crime Web sites. I especially like "Packaged Death," *Legal Studies Forum* 12, no. 2. See also http://tarlton.law.utexas.edu/lpop/etext/lsf/29-2/packaged.html and "The Molineux Case" on Jim Fisher's forensics Web site, http://jimfisher.edinboro.edu/forensics/mol1.html. Stories from the *New York Times* coverage of the case include: "Molineux Jury Complete," November 30, 1900, p. 3; "Molineux Murder Trial," January 6, 1900, p. 4; "Molineux's Next Ordeal," February 15, 1900, p. 12; "Molineux's Trial Progresses Rapidly," October 21, 1902, p. 1; "The Influences Acquitting Molineux," November 16, 1902, p. 11; "Tales From Jail," February 14, 1903, p. BR12; and the transcript of *New York v. Molineux,* appellant, Court of Appeals of New York, argued June 17, 1901, decided October 15, 1901, Opinion of the Court.

**Gettler had conducted a careful analysis . . . :** "Wood Alcohol Clue in Jackson Deaths," *New York Times,* April 29, 1922, p. 7.

**"the vilest concoctions masquerading . . .":** "Izzy, the Rum Hound, Tells How It's Done," *New York Times,* January 1, 1922, p. 3.

**Had the fumigator used hydrogen cyanide . . . :** The *New York Times* followed the Jackson case through the conclusion of the trial: "Thinks Fumigant Killed Jacksons," May 3, 1922, p. 10; "Rats in Poison Test May Solve Tragedy," May 4, 1922, p. 12; "2 Held for Deaths of Jackson Couple," May 9, 1922, p. 10; "Jury Frees Bradicich," August 3, 1922, p. 20; "Hotel Manager Cleared," December 13, 1922, p. 11.

**"In recent years, suicidal, accidental . . .":** Gettler and St. George, "Cyanide Poisoning."

**"should have made such inexcusable . . .":** Norris to Joseph Gallagher, assistant district attorney, Brooklyn, August 16, 1922; Norris to Gallagher, August 24, 1922, both in medical examiner's files, New York City Municipal Archive.

**Gettler also responded to the Bradicich trial . . . :** Alexander O. Gettler and J. Ogden Baine, "The Toxicology of Cyanide," *American Journal of the Medical Sciences* 195, no. 2, (February 1938), pp. 182–98.

**in 1980 the Hotel Margaret . . . :** Richard D. Lyons, "Work Starting on Embattled Site," *New York Times,* May 4, 1986.

## 4. Arsenic

**By early afternoon sixty people . . . :** "50 Ill of Poison Pie Eaten on Broadway," *New York Times,* August 1, 1922, p. 1; "Six Deaths Result From Arsenic Pie," *New York Times,* August 2, 1922, p. 1.

**The previous October, in an unnervingly similar incident . . . :** See "Poison Pie Clue in Similar Mystery," *New York Times,* August 8, 1922, p. 13.

**Years earlier Crones had worked . . . :** "Six Deaths Result from Poison Pie; Boasts of Poison Plot, Threatens Deaths in Letter," *New York Times,* February 17, 1916, p. 1; "Homicide in Chicago," http://homicide.northwestern.edu/context/timeline/1916/18/.

**Pure arsenic is a dark, grayish element . . . :** For history and background on arsenic, Witthaus and Becker, *Medical Jurisprudence,* pp. 4: 325–509, is a wonderfully detailed overview, from ancient history to Witthaus's experiments with taste, his attempts to gather data, and his amazingly gruesome descriptions of arsenic mummification. Emsley, *Elements of Murder,* pp. 141–69, offers a great survey of "arsenic murderers down the ages." Because of arsenic's prominent role in homicidal poisonings, it is found in every forensic science textbook in my bibliography, including both books produced by the New York City medical examiner's office.

**Charles Norris liked to get his hands bloody . . . :** The description of autopsy procedures at the medical examiner's office comes from Marten and Clarke, *Doctor Looks at Murder,* pp. 85–120; Milton Helpern, "The Postmortem Examination in Cases of Suspected Homicide," *Journal of Criminal Law and Criminology* 36, no. 6 (March–April 1946), pp. 485–522; Charles Norris, "The Medicolegal Necropsy," in *The Medicolegal Necropsy: A Symposium* (Baltimore: Williams & Wilkins Co., 1934), pp. 24–33.

**They'd interviewed the Shelbourne's owner . . . :** "Sure Poisoned Piece Was Meant to Kill," *New York Times,* August 3, 1922, p. 1.

**A major difficulty . . . :** W. A. Jackson, "To Die or Not to Dye: Poisoning from Arsenical Pigments in the Nineteenth Century," *Pharmaceutical History,* September 3, 1996, pp. 27–31; "Arsenics and Old Places," *Lancet,* July 8, 2000, p. 170; "Arsenic and Old Myths," *Rhode Island*

*Medicine,* July 1994, p. 234; Witthaus and Becker, *Medical Jurisprudence,* pp. 350–93.

**Racketeers across the United States . . . :** "Gunmen Shoot Six in East Side Swarm," *New York Times,* August 9, 1922, p. 1; "Nearly Pinch Izzy Chasing Rum Truck," *New York Times,* August 9, 1922, p. 13; "Gunman Kills Two," *New York Times,* August 12, 1922, p. 20.

**Even by federal estimates, two-thirds of the so-called "whiskey" . . . :** "Say Red Hook Carried 32 Percent Poison," *New York Times,* September 10, 1922, p. 20.

**Even in the tidy Brooklyn home . . . :** Gettler family interviews.

**"nothing of importance has been accomplished . . .":** A. O. Gettler, "On the Detection of Benzene in Cadavers," *Journal of Pharmacological Experimental Therapy* 21 (1923), pp. 161–64.

**Mary Frances Creighton, Fanny to her friends . . . :** "Creighton's Life Fight Today," *New York Daily News,* June 18, 1923, p. 1; "Death For Creightons Asked," *New York Daily News,* June 19, 1923, p. 1; "Dead Boy's Love Affair Denied," *New York Daily News,* June 19, 1923, p. 1; "Mrs. Creighton Faces Jury Calmly," *New*

*York Evening Post,* June 19, 1923, p.1; "Women Called in Creighton Poison Case," June 20, 1923, p. 1; "Try Woman for Killing Brother," *New York Evening Journal,* June 18, 1923, p.1; "Boy of 18 Murdered with Slow Poison," *New York Times,* May 13, 1923, p. 1; "To Exhume Bodies of the Creightons," *New York Times,* May 14, 1923, p. 3; "Dig Open Graves for Poison Clue," *New York Times,* May 16, 1923, p. 40; "Powdery Matter in Creighton Body," *New York Times,* May 19, 1923, p. 15; "Hints Young Avery Was a Poison Suicide," *New York Times,* May 20, 1923, p. 13; "Testifies to Poison in Body of Youth," *New York Times,* June 19, 1923, p. 11; "Creightons Freed of Murder Charge," *New York Times,* June 23, 1923, p. 13; "Mrs. Creighton Calm As New Trial Begins," *New York Times,* July 10, 1923, p. 40; "Creighton Defense to Rely on Experts," *New York Times,* July 13, 1923, p. 8; "Jury Again Acquits Mrs. Creighton of Murder Charge," *New York Times,* July 14, 1923, p. 1.

## 5. Mercury

**Ten months later his new wife was dead . . . :** "Rich Woman Dies in Biltmore Club; Poison Suspected," *New York*

*Times,* September 28, 1923, p. 1.

**"very much surprised when they heard . . .":** "Mrs. Webb Murdered With Slow Poison, Her Uncle Declares," *New York Times,* September 29, 1923, p. 1.

**Bichloride of mercury . . . :** Witthaus and Becker, *Medical Jurisprudence,* pp. 542–72, reviews the history of mercury poisonings, discussing elemental mercury and corrosive sublimate. See also Gonzales et al., *Pathology and Toxicology,* pp. 749–51; Peterson, Haines, and Webster, *Legal Medicine,* pp. 184–98; and Emsley, *Elements of Murder,* pp. 37–50. The Medline Plus online encyclopedia reviews the toxicity difference between elemental mercury and mercury salts: www.nlm.nih.gov/medlineplus/ency/article/002476.htm.

**The actress, Olive Thomas . . . :** Numerous Web sites detail the story of Olive Thomas. I like "The Life and Death of Olive Thomas" at www.public.asu.edu/~ialong/Taylor33.txt. It tells the story through newspaper and magazine clips, ranging from *Variety* and *Photoplay* to the *New York Telegraph.* Tim Lussier, "The Mysterious Death of Olive Thomas," is on the Silents Are Golden Web site at: www.silentsaregolden.com/articles/lpolivethomasdeath.html.

**"There is doubt . . .":** "Rich Woman Dies in Biltmore Club; Poison Suspected," *New York Times,* September 28, 1928, p. 1.

**He'd published his first paper on mercuric chloride . . . :** A. O. Gettler and A. V. St. George, "Suspected Case of Mercuric Chloride Poisoning," *Proceedings of the New York Pathological Society* 17, new series (1917), pp. 55–61. Gettler's work with the Reinsch test is described in Sidney Kaye, "The Rebirth and Blooming of Forensic Medicine," *American Journal of Forensic Medicine and Pathology* 13 (1992), p. 299; Peterson, Haines, and Webster, *Legal Medicine,* pp. 195–97.

**Well before Gertie Webb's organs arrived . . . :** Gonzales et al., *Pathology and Toxicology,* pp. 750–52.

**While she was still single . . . :** "Police Here Take Up Death of Mrs. Webb; Open Inquiry Today," *New York Times,* October 1, 1923, p. 1; "Webb Is Questioned About Wife's Death; Trace Poison Found," *New York Times,* October 2, 1923, p. 1; "Webb Offers Aid in Death Mystery; Knows of No Poison," *New York Times,* October 3, 1923, p. 1.

**The Westchester district attorney's office . . . :** "Mercury Revealed in Mrs.

Webb's Body by Chemical Test," *New York Times,* October 4, 1923, p. 1; "Not Enough Poison to Cause Her Death in Mrs. Webb's Body," *New York Times,* October 5, 1923, p. 1; "Sudden New Turn in Webb Mystery Is Now Expected," *New York Times,* October 8, 1923, p. 1; "To Exonerate Webb in a Report Today," *New York Times,* October 19, 1923, p. 6; "Jury Clears Webb in Death of Wife," *New York Times,* October 21, 1923, p. 1.

**the death of the famous Blue Man . . . :** A. O. Gettler, C. P. Rhoades, and Soma Weiss, "A Contribution to the Pathology of Generalized Argyria with a Discussion on the Fate of Silver in the Human Body," *American Journal of Pathology* 3 (1927), pp. 631–61.

**Charles Webb was still fighting with his dead wife's family . . . :** "Relatives Attack Mrs. Webb's Will," *New York Times,* December 11, 1923, p. 18; "Webb Wins on Will by Order of Court," *New York Times,* December 12, 1923, p. 1; "Surrogate Upholds Will of Mrs. Webb," *New York Times,* December 23, 1923, p. E1; "Webb Kin Claim House and $250,000," *New York Times,* July 16, 1924, p. 36.

**It began in the Standard Oil Refin-**

ery . . . : "Odd Gas Kills One, Makes Four Insane," *New York Times,* October 27, 1924, p. 1; "Third Victim Dies From Poison Gas," *New York Times,* October 29, 1924, p. 3; "Bar Ethyl Gasoline As 5th Victim Dies," *New York Times,* October 30, 1924, p. 1.

**Tetraethyl lead — or TEL, in industrial shorthand . . . :** Background on the use of TEL in gasoline and the inventor Thomas Midgley Jr. (who also developed Freon) can be found at "Thomas Midgley's Dubious Legacy," http://expertvoices.nsdl.org/highlights/2008/03/17/thomas-midgleys-dubious-legacy/. For a different perspective, see Invent Now's Hall of Fame, at www.invent.org/hall_of_fame/193.html.

**The statement failed to impress the State of New Jersey . . . :** "Stops Jersey Sale of Ethyl Gasoline," *New York Times,* November 4, 1924, p. 37.

**"The fact that it is readily absorbed . . .":** "Tetraethyl Lead in Victim's Brain," *New York Times,* November 13, 1924; "Nine of DuPont Plant Died," *New York Times,* November 2, 1924, p. 22.

**"I'm taking no chances whatever . . .":** "Another Man Dies from Insanity Gas," *New York Times,* October 28, 1924, p. 25.

**It took Gettler a full three weeks . . . :**
Alexander O. Gettler and Charles Norris,
"Poisoning by Tetra-ethyl Lead: Postmortem and Clinical Findings," *Journal of the
American Medical Association,* 8 (1925),
pp. 818–20; "Report Condemns Making
of Lead Gas," *New York Times,* November
27, 1925, p. 14.

**After Norris released his office's re-
port . . . :** William Kovarik, "Ethyl: The
1920s Environmental Conflict Over
Leaded Gasoline and Alternative Fuels," a
paper given to the American Society for
Environmental History, Providence,
Rhode Island, March 26–30, 2003,
www.radford.edu/~wkovarik/papers/
ethylconflict.html; Jamie Lincoln Kitman,
"The Secret History of Lead," *Nation* 270
(March 20, 2000), www.thenation.com/
doc/20000320/kitman.

**"its use should be prohibited, for
lead . . .":** Norris to Frank. J. Monoghan,
health commissioner, November 14, 1924,
medical examiner's files, New York City
Municipal Archive.

**That same May, a twenty-one-year-old
White Plains woman . . . :** "Grand-
mother Held as Girl's Poisoner," *New York
Times,* May 24, 1925, p. 25.

**"we have been swamped with unknown**

**floaters . . .":** Norris to John T. Walsh, Department of Health, May 19, 1925, medical examiner's files, New York City Municipal Archive.

**In July he decided to take his first vacation . . . :** Norris to Hylan, June 5, 1925, medical examiner's files, New York City Municipal Archive.

**Rich enough, though . . . :** "Webb Gross Estate Set at $1,0333,765," *New York Times,* July 21, 1928, p. 26.

**Webb donated the empty plot she'd owned . . . :** "Webb Gives Tract to City for Park," *New York Times,* June 21, 1929, p. 29; "City Accepts Playground," *New York Times,* April 24, 1930, p. 31; "Gorman Park," New York City Department of Parks and Recreation, www.nycgovparks.org/parks/M031/highlights/12328.

## 6. Carbon Monoxide

**In late January 1926 . . . :** "Noisiest Spot Here, Sixth Avenue At 34th Street," *New York Times,* January 16, 1926, p. 7.

**"Let the people know that selfishness . . .":** Hylan to Norris, May 24, 1924, medical examiner's files, New York City Municipal Archive.

**"I understand that the taxicabs . . .":** Norris to Albert Goldman, commissioner of plants and structures, January 4, 1926; Goldman to Norris, January 15, 1926; both in medical examiner's files, New York City Municipal Archive.

**In 1920 the medical examiner's office tallied . . . :** "Demand State Curb to End Auto Deaths," *New York Times,* October 7, 1922.

**"constitute a menace to the general public . . .":** "Report No Danger in Ethyl Gasoline," *New York Times,* January 20, 1925, p. 13.

**the main by-product is carbon dioxide . . . :** Marten, *Doctor Looks at Murder,* pp. 246–59; Peterson, Haines, and Webster, *Legal Medicine,* pp. 293–96.

**"This brings up a rather interesting . . .":** Marten, "Asphyxia," p. 260.

**On the other hand, carbon monoxide . . . :** Witthaus and Becker, *Medical Jurisprudence,* pp. 4: 847–50; Dieter Pankow, "History of Carbon Monoxide Toxicology," in David G. Penney, ed., *Carbon Monoxide Toxicity* (Boca Raton, Fla.: CRC Press, 2000), pp. 1–17; "Carbon Monoxide as an Unrecognized Cause of Neurasthenia: A History," ibid., pp. 231–55.

**Charles Norris estimated that carbon monoxide . . . :** "5,581 Deaths in 1925

Classed as Violent," *New York Times,* October 19, 1926, p. 29.

**An out-of-work painter named Harry Freindlich . . . :** Alexander O. Gettler, "The Historical Development of Toxicology," presented at the annual meeting of the American Academy of Forensic Sciences, Chicago, February 26–28, 1953, pp. 9–10; Gettler, "Toxicology in the Medicolegal Necropsy," in Magath, *Medicolegal Necropsy,* pp. 60–61; "Wife Smothered Then Gas Turned On," *New York Times,* November 14, 1923, p. 8.

**Carbon monoxide can be considered as a kind of chemical thug . . . :** Harrison S. Martland, "Medical Examiners' Findings in Deaths from Shooting, Stabbing, Cutting and Asphyxia," in Magath, *Medicolegal Necropsy,* pp. 143–47; Hendrik J. Vreman, Ronald J. Wong, and David K. Stevenson, "Carbon Monoxide in Breath, Blood and Other Tissues," in Penney, *Carbon Monoxide Toxicity,* pp. 19–61.

**In Alexander Gettler's laboratory, one of the simplest ways . . . :** "Carbon Monoxide," in Peterson, Haines, and Webster, *Legal Medicine,* pp. 296–324; Gonzales, Vance, and Helpern, *Legal Medicine and Toxicology,* pp. 496–521, 956–59.

**During his first month in office . . . :**

"Accidental Deaths by Illuminating Gas During Month of January 1918," medical examiner's files, New York City Municipal Archive.

**In 1925 the details . . . :** "Fifteen Are Killed by Gas in One Day," *New York Times,* January 27, 1925, p. 3.

**"the public generally does not . . .":** "Mine Bureau Warns of Dangers in Gas," *New York Times,* August 26, 1928, p. 20.

**could carbon monoxide be absorbed after death?:** Alexander O. Gettler and Henry C. Freimuth, "The Carbon Monoxide Content of the Blood Under Various Conditions," *American Journal of Clinical Pathology* 11 (1940), pp. 603–16.

**In October 1926 Norris issued his yearly analysis . . . :** "5,581 Deaths in 1925 Classed as Violent," *New York Times,* October 19, 1926, p. 29.

**In the first week of that foggy month . . . :** "Slayer Is Caught Disposing of Limbs," *New York Times,* December 1, 1926, p. 29; "Police Capture Man Toting Hacked Body," *New York Daily News,* December 3, 1926, p. 1; Frank J. Jirka, *American Doctors of Destiny* (Chicago: Normandie House, 1940), pp. 216–29; "Murder Trial Interrupted," *New York Times,* March 16, 1927, p. 17; "Acquitted of Murder, Held on New Charge," *New York Times,* March 18, 1927, p. 7.

## 7. Methyl Alcohol

**The rumors began . . . :** "Says Alcohol Deaths Will Soon Increase," *New York Times,* August 3, 1926, p. 22; "Defend Poisons Put Into Alcohol," *New York Times,* August 11, 1926, p. 23; "Under Way," *Time,* August 23, 1926, www.time.com/time/magazine/article/ 0.9171.729415.00.html; "New Denaturant for Alcohol Near," *New York Times,* September 4, 1926, p. 28; "Drop Two Recipes for Trade Alcohol," *New York Times,* September 11, 1926, p. 6; "Government to Double Alcohol Poison Content and Also Add Benzene," *New York Times,* December 30, 1926, p. 1.

**As the year pulled toward its close . . . :** "23 Deaths Here Laid to Holiday Drinking; 89 Ill in Hospitals," *New York Times,* December 28, 1926, p. 1.

**"The government knows":** Ibid.

**"in the same category as the man . . .":** "Poisonous Alcohol Stays for Present, Mellon Tells Drys," *New York Times,* December 29, 1926, p. 1.

**Nicholas Murray Butler:** "Dr. Butler Against Prohibition Cause," *New York*

*Times,* February 12, 1927, p. 13; "Says Butler Shows a Yellow Streak," February 13, 1927, p. 21.

**The pathologists and chemists . . . :** "Poison Rum Toll Continues to Rise," *New York Times,* January 1, 1927, p. 5; "Government Won't Drop Poison Alcohol Policy; Deaths Here 400 in Year," *New York Times,* January 1; 1927, p. 1; " 'Murder' by Poison Bootleg Liquor," *Literary Digest,* January 15, 1927, p. 1; "Most of Our Liquor Poison, 741 Deaths in City in 1926, Norris Reports to Walker," *New York Times,* February 6, 1927, p. 1; "Dr. Norris's Poison Liquor Report," *Literary Digest,* February 26, 1927, p. 14.

**a warning that German methanol . . . :** "Warns There Is Death in Drinking Methanol," *New York Times,* April 30, 1925, p. 7.

**a law to halt the extra poisoning of industrial alcohol . . . :** "Poison," *Time,* January 10, 1927, www.time.com/time/magazine/article/0.9171.881577.00.html; "Wets Plan Fight over Denaturants," *New York Times,* January 2, 1927, p. 3; "Congress Wets Denounce Deaths by Poison Alcohol as Government Murders," *New York Times,* January 4, 1927, p. 1; "Senate

Calls on Mellon to Tell Part Drys Played in Fixing Poison Alcohol," *New York Times,* January 5, 1927, p. 1; "Congress Requires Poison in Alcohol, Mellon Declares," *New York Times,* January 12, 1927.

**The complicated murder of Albert Snyder . . . :** The story of Ruth Snyder and Judd Gray is told in Landis MacKellar, *The "Double Indemnity" Murder* (Syracuse: N.Y.: Syracuse University Press, 2006), and is featured on numerous crime websites, including "The Dumb Bell Murder," Dead Men Do Tell Tales, www.prairie ghosts.com/ruth_judd.html, and "The Snyder-Gray Murder Case, Part 1," www.trivia-library.com/a/the-snyder-gray-murder-case-part-1.htm, and "The Snyder-Gray Murder Case, Part 2," www.trivia-library.com/a/the-snyder-gray-murder-case-part-2.html. James Cain's use of the case in his novels is discussed in an essay on *The Postman Always Rings Twice* at www.swisseduc.ch/english/reading list/cain_james/postman/background.html.

**In March 1927 Ruth and Albert Snyder . . . :** Coverage in *New York Times* includes "Slayers Indicted; Snyder Case Trial Sought for April 4," March 24, 1927, p. 1; "Poisoned Whisky in Snyder Home Bares Early Plot," March 25, 1927, p.1;

"Poison a Mystery in the Snyder Case," March 28, 1927, p. 1; "State Builds Case in Snyder Murder," April 3, 1927, p. 12; "Mrs. Snyder Breaks As Trial Day Nears," April 17, 1927, p. 1; "Full Snyder Jury Picked on Fifth Day; Trial On Monday," April 23, 1927, p. 1; "Snyder Jury Hears Gray's Confession Accusing Woman," April 28, 1927, p. 1; "Child to Testify After Mrs. Snyder Faces State's Fire," May 1, 1927, p. 10; "Gray Denies Wish to Kill; Insists Woman Dominated; Jury May Get Case Today," May 6, 1927, p. 12; "Gray and Woman Make Last Appeals to the Jury Today," May 9, 1927, p. 1; "Courts Refusal to Permit Controversy Sped Case to a Verdict in Eleven Days," May 10, 1927, p. 21.

**Ruby Gonzales . . . :** "Two Physicians Arrested," *New York Times,* September 16, 1927, p. 25; "Deny Causing Woman's Death," *New York Times,* September 17, 1927, p. 19; "Dr. Eisenberg is Convicted," *New York Times,* April 18, 1928, p. 18.

**how long did it take for chloroform to leave a brain? . . . :** A. O. Gettler and H. Blume, "Chloroform Content of the Brain Following Anesthesia," *Archives of Pathology and Laboratory Medicine* 11 (1931), pp. B41–53; A. O. Gettler and

H. Blume, "Chloroform Content of Brain, Lungs and Liver: Quantitative Recovery and Determination," *Archives of Pathology and Laboratory Medicine* 11 (1931), pp. 554–60.

**The scene around the high walls . . . :** "She Goes to Death First," *New York Times,* January 13, 1928, p. 1; David J. Kracijek, *Scooped!* (New York: Columbia University Press, 1999), p. 90.

## 8. Radium

**Harrison Stanford Martland:** Harrison Martland's papers are archived at the University of Medicine and Dentistry of New Jersey Library Special Collections. His biography is posted at the main Web address for the Martland Collection, www.umdnj.edu/librweb/speccoll/Mart land.html, which also reviews his research projects in occupational health.

**The French physicist Henri Becquerel . . . :** "Marie and Pierre Curie and the Discovery of Polonium and Radium," at Nobelprize.org.

**There were bottles of radium water . . . :** Roger M. Macklis, "The Great Radium Scandal," *Scientific American,* August 1993, pp. 94–99.

**a peculiar health crisis in Orange, New**

Jersey . . . : The story of the dial painters' illnesses is told in the context of
industrial health reform in Claudia Clark,
*Radium Girls* (Chapel Hill: University of
North Carolina Press, 1997) and in terms
of toxicology in Harrison S. Martland and
Robert E. Humphries, "Osteogenic Sar-
coma in Dial Painters Using Luminous
Paint," *Archives of Pathology and Laboratory Medicine* 7 (1929), pp. 406–11.

**As Curie demonstrated . . . :** "Radium
Gift Awaits Mme. Curie Here," *New York
Times,* February 27, 1921, p. 10; "How
Mme. Curie Discovered Radium," *New
York Times,* February 27, 1921, p. 7;
"Mme. Curie Sails May 7," *New York
Times,* March 31, 1921, p. E1; "Mme.
Curie's Genius," *New York Times,* May 10,
1921, p. 88.

**The women were exhaling radon gas
. . . :** Harrison S. Martland, Philip Con-
lon, and Joseph P. Knef, "Some Unrecognized Dangers in the Use and Handling
of Radioactive Substances," *Journal of the
American Medical Association,* December
5, 1925, p. 1769; Harrison S. Martland,
"Microscopic Changes of Certain Anemias Due to Radioactivity," *Archives of
Pathology and Laboratory Medicine* 6

(October 1926), pp. 465–72; Gonzales, Vana, and Helpern, *Legal Medicine and Toxicology,* pp. 757–59.

**The bones belonged to an Italian-American, Amelia Maggia . . . :** "Body to Be Exhumed in Radium Poison Test," *New York Times,* October 10, 1927, p. 9; Irving Sunshine, "Dr. Alexander O. Gettler's Documentation of a Radiation Hazard," *American Journal of Forensic Medicine and Pathology* 4, no. 4 (December 1983), pp. 307–09; A. V. St. George, Alexander O. Gettler, and Ralph H. Muller, "Radioactive Substances in a Body Five Years After Death," *Archives of Pathology and Laboratory Medicine* 7 (1929), pp. 397–405.

**As the lawsuit dragged on, the five Radium Girls . . . :** Harrison S. Martland, "Occupational Poisoning in Manufacture of Luminous Watch Dials," *Journal of the American Medical Association* 92, no. 6 (February 9, 1929), pp. 466–73; Bill Kavarik, "The Radium Girls," www.runet.edu/~wkovarik/envhist/radium .html; "Women Ask $1,250,000 in Radium Poisoning; Hear in Court Their Chance to Live Is Slender," *New York Times,* April 27, 1928, p. 1; "5 Radium

Suits Set for Trial on June 8," *New York Times,* May 20, 1928, p. 7; "Moves to Settle Five Radium Suits," June 1, 1928, p. 10.

**"They all say 'Why pick on us . . .' ":** *"Rogers' Tip to Speculators: Don't Sell Democrats Short," New York Times,* June 5, 1928, p. 31.

**The first October weekend, four New Yorkers were killed . . . :** "Four Dead, 18 Ill of Poison Liquor," *New York Times,* October 3, 1928, p. 11; "11 Dead, 60 Ill in Day Is City Liquor Toll," *New York Times,* October 8, 1928, p. 1; "20 Speakeasies Raided in Drive Backed by Mayor as Liquor Kills 29 in Day," *New York Times,* October 9, 1928, p. 1.

**In October 1929, Marie Curie made another radium tour . . . :** "Marie Curie Is Guest of Friends in Country," *New York Times,* October 17, 1929, p. 29; "Mme. Curie to Get Medal," *New York Times,* October 21, 1929, p. 16; "Mme. Curie at White House," *New York Times,* October 30, 1929, p. 21; "Mme. Curie Receives $50,000 Radium Gift," *New York Times,* October 31, 1929, p. 1.

**J. J. Riordan, head of the County Trust Company . . . :** Marten, *Doctor Looks at*

*Murder,* pp. 47–49.

## 9. Ethyl Alcohol

**"Case 1: A moderate drinker . . .":** Alexander O. Gettler, "A Study of the Alcoholic Content of Autopsy Material, and Its Bearing on the Cause of Death," *Bulletin of the New York Academy of Medicine* 4, no. 6 (June 1928), pp. 715–27.

**"From almost every standpoint ethyl alcohol . . .":** Alexander O. Gettler and Arthur Tiber, "The Alcoholic Content of the Human Brain," *Archives of Pathology and Laboratory Medicine* 3 (1927), pp. 218–26.

**In early 1930 the Metropolitan Life Insurance** . . . : "Alcohol Deaths Up 300 Percent Since 1920," *New York Times,* October 23, 1930, p. 28; "Dry Conflict Acute After 10-Year Test," *New York Times,* January 1, 1930, p. 3.

**The primary alcohols, including methyl and ethyl, . . . :** Gonzales et al., *Pathology and Toxicology,* pp. 781–85; Peterson, Haines, and Webster, *Legal Medicine,* pp. 614–32; www.chemguide.co.uk/organic props/alcohols/background.html; William Boggan, Ph.D., "Alcohol and You," General Chemistry Case Studies, www.chem cases.com/alcohol/index.html.

**No one had figured out how much alcohol in the blood meant intoxication . . . :** Alexander O. Gettler and A.W. Freireich, "The Nature of Alcohol Tolerance," *Forensic Medicine,* February 1925, pp. 328–33.

**"Mama cried out and said . . .":** Dan Baum, "Jake Leg," *New Yorker,* September 15, 2003, pp. 50–57 and "The Jake Walk Blues: A Toxicologic Tragedy Mirrored in American Popular Music," *Annals of Internal Medicine* 84, no. 6 (December 1976), 804–808. See also A. D. Woolf, "Ginger Jake and the Blues: A Tragic Song of Poisoning," *Veterinary and Human Toxicology* 37, no. 3 (June 1995), pp. 252–54.

**From Brooklyn arose another . . . :** "Arrested as Maker of Deadly Drink," *New York Times,* May 1, 1930, p. 5.

**It took months for scientists to identify the plasticizer . . . :** "Paralyzing Drink Has Carbolic Acid," *New York Times,* March 29, 1930, p. 6; " 'Ginger Jake' Is a Puzzle," *New York Times,* July 13, 1930, p. 13.

**the chemist had purchased perfumes . . . :** "Kansas Ginger Jury Indicts Firms Here," *New York Times,* July 30, 1930, p. 5.

**By 1930, Gettler had assembled an**

**encyclopedic list . . . :** Gettler and Tiber, "Alcoholic Content"; Alexander O. Gettler, Joseph B. Niederl, and A. A. Benedetti-Pichler, "The Isolation of Pure, Anhydrous Ethyl Alcohol from Non-Alcoholic Human and Animal Tissues," *Journal of the American Chemical Society* 54, no. 4 (April 6, 1932), pp. 1476–85; Alexander O. Gettler and A. Walter Freireich, "Determination of Alcoholic Intoxication During Life by Spinal Fluid Analysis," *Journal of Biological Chemistry* 92 (1931), pp. 199–209.

**another twenty were dead in Newark . . . :** "20th Newark Death Gives Alcohol Clue," *New York Times,* October 15, 1930, p. 17.

**"a certain type of person with uncontrollable . . .":** Doran made his comments in the context of another attempt by "wet" politicians to force the government to stop adding extra poisons to industrial alcohol. Like earlier attempts, that effort failed: "Wets Are Defeated in First House Test on Balking Dry Law," *New York Times,* December 6, 1930, p. 1; "Poison Alcohol Takes Larger Toll," *New York Times,* December 19, 1930, p. 1.

**seemingly able to guzzle alcohol without obvious effect . . . :** A. O. Gettler and

H. Freireich, "The Nature of Alcohol Tolerance," *Forensic Medicine,* February 1935, pp. 328–34.

**In his annual report, issued that spring . . . :** "6,525 Fatalities in City Last Year," *New York Times,* May 19, 1931, p. 14.

**"At the present time I am spending nearly . . .":** Norris to Charles F. Kerrigan, assistant mayor, February 10, 1932, medical examiner's files, New York City Municipal Archive.

**"told me that this disease is an obscure one . . .":** Harrison Martland, "The Occurrence of Malignancy in Radioactive Persons," *American Journal of Cancer Research* 15, no. 4, (1931), pp. 2435–516.

**Here was an "important" radium death . . . :** Roger M. Macklis, "The Great Radium Scandal," *Scientific American,* August 1993, p. 99; R. M. Macklis, "Radithor and the Era of Mild Radiation Therapy," *Journal of the American Medical Association* 264, no. 5 (August 1, 1990), http://jama.ama-assn.org/cgi/content/abstract/264/5/614.

**Eben M. Byers was chairman of . . . :** "Eben M. Byers Dies of Radium Poisoning," *New York Times,* April 1, 1932, p. 1; "Death Stirs Action on Radium Cures,"

*New York Times,* April 2, 1932, p. 12; "Doctors Seek Ban on Radium Water," *New York Times,* May 12, 1932, p. 3; Alexander O. Gettler and Charles Norris, "Poisoning from Drinking Radium Water," *Journal of the American Medical Association,* February 11, 1933, pp. 400–403.

**The new crisis resulted from an administration change . . . :** Norris to McKee, September 19, 1932, medical examiner's files, New York City Municipal Archive; "McKee Says Bankers Force Budget Cuts; Dr. Norris Resigns," *New York Times,* September 21, 1932, p. 1; "Norris Quits Post as Chief Examiner," *New York Times,* September 21, 1932, p. 3; "Doctors Urge McKee to Ask Norris to Stay," *New York Times,* September 24, 1932, p. 2; "Dr. Norris Returns as City Medical Examiner; Withdraws Resignation at the Mayor's Behest," *New York Times,* September 28, 1932, p. 1; "Post Mortem," *Time,* October 3, 1932, www.time.com/time/magazine/article/0,9171,744511,00.html.

**The news was, for a change, unusually good . . . :** "Only Two Deaths Laid to Poison Liquor," *New York Times,* December 27, 1932, p. 2.

## 10. Carbon Monoxide

**a dusty little store that never seemed to open . . . :** This description is based on a photo published in the *New York Daily News* in 1933 and reprinted in Simon Read, *On the House: The Bizarre Killing of Michael Malloy* (New York: Berkley Books, 2005). Read's book provided background for the Malloy story, along with "The Indestructible Man," in Richard Glyn Jones, ed., *Poison!* (New York: Berkley Books, 1987), pp. 58–71; Marshall Houts, *Where Death Delights* (New York: Coward-McCann, 1967), pp. 125–38.

**On February 20, Congress voted to repeal . . . :** See David J. Hanson, "Repeal of Prohibition in the U.S.," www2.potsdam.edu/hansondj/controversies/1131637220.html; and Marvin Hintz, *Farewell, John Barleycorn: Prohibition in the United States* (Minneapolis: Lerner Publications, 1996).

**"Case 2: Male, age 38, found dead . . .":** A. O. Gettler and H. C. Freimuth, "Carbon Monoxide in Blood," *American Journal of Clinical Pathology* 13, no. 79 (1943), pp. 10–17.

**In April 1933 legal beer . . . :** "Brewers Here Swamped," *New York Times,* April 8, 1933, p. 1; "Thirsty Throngs Jam City

Streets," *New York Times,* April 8, 1933, p. 2.

**Too many were willing to share their part . . . :** "Insurance Murder Charged to Five," *New York Times,* May 13, 1933, p. 1; "Murder Plot Seen in Another Death," *New York Times,* May 14, 1933, p. 27; "Murder Inquiry Is Widened by Foley," *New York Times,* May 16, 1933, p. 18; "Indicted as Slayers in Insurance Plot," *New York Times,* May 17, 1933, p. 8.

**the formation of a new department:** forensic medicine . . . : "NYU Will Train Medical Officers," *New York Times,* June 11, 1933, p. N4; "Science and Crime," *New York Times,* June 18, 1933, p. E4: "Program Outline and Requirements," unpublished document, 1933, medical examiner's files, New York City Municipal Archive.

**"The clerks seem to think an undertaker . . .":** Edward F. Donovan, funeral director, to Charles Norris, March 7, 1933, medical examiner's files, New York City Municipal Archive.

**"A great deal of the trouble . . .":** Norris to George Goodstein, May 13, 1933, medical examiner's files, New York City Municipal Archive.

**Prohibition might still be . . . :** "July Thirst Sets 3.2 Beer Record," *New York Times,* September 1, 1933, p. 36.

**Smokers could choose from among almost three hundred . . . :** Emil Bogen, "The Composition of Cigarets and Cigaret Smoke," *Journal of the American Medical Association* (October 12, 1929), pp. 1110–14.

**"headaches experienced by heavy smokers . . .":** A. O. Gettler and M. R. Mattice, " 'Normal' Carbon Monoxide Content of the Blood," *Journal of the American Medical Association* 100, no. 92 (January 14, 1933), pp. 92–97.

**Nicotine is a naturally occurring . . . :** Thorwald, *Century of the Detective,* pp. 296–307; Peterson, Haines, and Webster, *Legal Toxicology,* pp. 554–65; Gonzales et al., *Pathology and Toxicology,* pp. 844–45, 1140–42; "Case Definition: Nicotine Poisoning," U.S. Centers for Disease Control, www.bt.cdc.gov/agent/nicotine/casedef.asp.

**an analysis done in 1929 pointed out that tobacco plants . . . :** Bogen, "Composition of Cigarets."

**They'd also found cyanide, hydrogen sulfide, . . . :** Ibid.; W. E. Dixon, "The Tobacco Habit," *Lancet,* October 22,

1927, pp. 881–85; "Is Tobacco Smoke Carbon Monoxide Eliminating the 'Red-Blooded' Man?," *New York Times,* November 7, 1926, p. X16.

**The durability of carbon monoxide in a dead body . . . :** A. O. Gettler and H. C. Freimuth, "Carbon Monoxide in Blood," *American Journal of Clinical Pathology* 13, no. 99 (1943), pp. 79–83; "The Carbon Monoxide Content of Blood Under Various Conditions," *American Journal of Clinical Pathology* 10 (1940), pp. 603–16.

**And Mike Malloy's blood? . . . :** "Four on Trial in Bronx Insurance Slaying," *New York Times,* October 5, 1933, p. 16; "Jury Weighs Fate of Four in Killing," *New York Times,* October 19, 1933, p. 42; "Four Men to Die for Bronx Killing," *New York Times,* October 20, 1933, p. 38.

**In Manhattan, as the clock ticked away . . . :** "Chefs Jubilant at Dry Law Doom," *New York Times,* November 11, 1933, p. 1.

**Utah, the last state needed to complete . . . :** "City Toasts New Era," *New York Times,* December 6, 1933, p. 1.

**On June 3, 1934, Tony Marino, Frank Pasqua, . . . :** "Three Die at Sing Sing for Bronx Murder," *New York Times,* June

8, 1934, p. 44; "Murphy Goes to the Chair," *New York Times,* July 6, 1934, p. 10; Robert Campbell, "Three Die in Chair for Barfly Murder," *New York Daily Mirror,* June 8, 1934, p. 1.

## 11. Thallium

**There were times, and they came frequently enough . . . :** Arthur Kallet and F. J. Schlink, *100,000,000 Guinea Pigs: Dangers in Everyday Foods, Drugs and Cosmetics* (New York: Grosset and Dunlap, 1935); Ruth De Forest Lamb, *American Chamber of Horrors: The Truth About Food and Drugs* (New York: Grosset and Dunlap, 1936).

**The depilatory creams had created a small but significant epidemic . . . :** "Dangers from Use of Thallium Acetate," *Journal of the American Medical Association* 94, no. 2 (January 18, 1931), p. 197; "Thallium Poisoning," *Journal of the American Medical Association* 95, no. 3 (January 30, 1932), pp. 406–407; "A Case of Thallium Poisoning Following the Prolonged Use of a Depilatory Cream," *Journal of the American Medical Association* 96, no. 22 (March 30, 1933), pp. 1866–68; "Reports of Thallium Acetate Poisoning Following Use of Koremlu [a depila-

tory cream made in New York City],"
*Journal of the American Medical Association,* 1868–69; William Mahoney, "Retrobulbar Neuritis Due to Thallium Poisoning from Depilatory Cream," *Journal of the American Medical Association* 98, no. 8 (February 20, 1932), pp. 618–20.

**He was such a nice man . . . :** "Five in Family Killed by a Rare Poison; Father Is Accused," *New York Times,* May 11, 1935, p. 1; "Five Poisonings Denied by Father in Court; No Motive Is Found," *New York Times,* May 12, 1935, p. 1.

**The name *thallium* comes from the Greek . . . :** Emsley, *Elements of Murder,* "Thallium: The Essentials," www.webelements.com/thallium/; Jefferson Lab, "It's Elemental," http://education.jlab.org/itselemental/ele081.html; "Thallium: Statistics and Information," http://minerals.usgs.gov/minerals/pubs/commodity/thallium/.

**"its relatively rare occurrence . . .":** Louis Weiss, *A Study of Thallium Poisoning,* Ph.D. diss., New York University, 1942.

**As the U.S. Public Health Service noted in a review . . . :** Francis Heyroth, *Thallium: A Review and Summary of Medical Literature,* Supplement No. 197 to the

Public Health Reports (Washington, D.C.: United States Government Printing Office, 1947).

**As state wildlife officials discovered . . . :** Jean M. Linsdale, "Facts Concerning the Use of Thallium in California to Poison Rodents: Its Destructiveness to Game Birds, Song Birds and Other Valuable Wildlife," *Condor* 33, no. 3 (May–June 1931), pp. 92–106.

**"In subacute cases, where the patient lives . . .":** Alexander O. Gettler and Louis Weiss, "Thallium Poisoning I: The Detection of Thallium in Biologic Material," *American Journal of Clinical Pathology* 13 (1943), pp. 322–26; Gonzales et al., *Pathology and Toxicology,* pp. 756–57.

**Surely, the Brooklyn detectives thought, . . . :** "New Clues Found in Poisoning of Five," *New York Times,* May 13, 1935, p. 1; "Thallium Is Found in Gross Cocoa Can," *New York Times,* May 13, 1935, p. 1.

**"So far we have uncovered nothing . . .":** "Prosecutor Hints at Freeing Gross," *New York Times,* May 15, 1935, p. 44.

**In cases of thallium poisoning, autopsy results . . . :** Alexander O. Gettler and Louis Weiss, "Thallium Poisoning III:

Clinical Toxicology of Thallium," *American Journal of Clinical Pathology* 13 (1943), pp. 422–29.

**The chemical tests for thallium were an intricate . . . :** Gettler and Weiss, "Thallium Poisoning I."

**Further, repeated analyses of the cocoa found . . . :** "Gross Cocoa Found Free of Thallium," *New York Times,* May 18, 1935, p. 3.

**On May 20, a Brooklyn magistrate . . . :** "Gross Is Released in Poison Deaths," *New York Times,* May 21, 1935, p. 40.

**"Let your voice be heard loudly . . .":** Kallet and Schlink, *100,000,000 Guinea Pigs,* p. 302.

**Elixir Sulfanilamide . . . :** U.S. Food and Drug Administration, "Taste of Raspberries, Taste of Death: The 1937 Elixir Sulfanilamide Incident," www.fda.gov/oc/history/elixir.html; Paul Wax, "Elixirs, Diluents, and the Passage of the 1938 Food, Drug and Cosmetics Act," *Annals of Internal Medicine* 122, no. 6 (March 15, 1995), pp. 456–61.

**"I am avoiding going out . . .":** Norris to Philip Hoerter, Detectives' Endowment Association, April 15, 1935, medical examiner's files, New York City Municipal Archive.

**"You ask me how I am . . .":** Norris to Charles Miller, Yale Alumni University Fund Association, April 17, 1935, medical examiner's files, New York City Municipal Archive.

**The commission calculated that 40 percent . . . :** "Graft of $170,000 in 'Fees' Charged to Aides of Norris," *New York Times,* May 27, 1935, p. 1.

**Within a month a formal investigation . . . :** "Blanshard Clears Aides of Dr. Norris," *New York Times,* June 28, 1935, p. 23.

**On the morning of September 11 . . . :** "Dr. Norris, 67, Dies of Sudden Illness," *New York Times,* September 12, 1935, p. 1; "Dr. Norris Buried with High Honors," *New York Times,* September 15, 1935, p. 38; "Dr. Norris Set Up Trust for Wife," *New York Times,* September 21, 1935, p. 13.

**The staff took up a collection . . . :** "Receipts and Expenditures — Portrait (Painting) of Dr. Charles Norris," September 1936, medical examiner's files, New York City Municipal Archives.

**"because of the great friendship . . .":** Thomas Gonzales to Mendel Jacobi, July 23, 1936, medical examiner's files, New York City Municipal Archive.

**"In sending my small contribution . . .":** Mendel Jacobi to Thomas Gonzales, July 21, 1936, medical examiner's files, New York City Municipal Archive.

**The case began in mid-September . . . :** On the Creighton-Appelgate murder case, see, Leonard Gribble, "The Long Island Borgia," in Richard Glyn Jones, ed., *Poison!* (New York: Berkley Books, 1987), pp. 100–12; Dorothy Kilgallen, *Murder One* (New York: Random House, 1967); *The People of the State of New York, Respondent v. Frances Q. Creighton and Everett C. Appelgate, Appellants,* Court of Appeals of New York, 271 N.Y. 263; 2 N.E. 2nd 650; 1936; and the following newspaper accounts: "Find Poison Enough to Kill 3 in Wife's Body; Quiz Husband," *New York Daily News,* October 7, 1935, p. 1; "Wife Dead by Poison, Quiz Mate," *New York Post,* October 7, 1935, p. 1; "Woman Confesses Arsenic Slaying," *New York Times,* October 9, 1935, p. 1; "Admits She Poisoned Friend and Own Kin," *New York Daily News,* October 9, 1935, p. 1; "State Maps Case to Send Mrs. Creighton to Chair," *New York Evening Journal,* October 10, 1935, p. 1; "Ruth Creighton Refuses to Save Lover at Altar," *New York Daily*

*News,* October 10, 1935, p. 2; "Suspected Borgia, Kin Asserts," *New York Daily Mirror,* October 11, 1935, p. 1; "Indict Appelgate, Mrs. Creighton," *New York Post,* October 11, 1935, p. 1; "Husband Indicted in Arsenic Murder," *New York Times,* October 12, 1935, p. 2; "Mrs. Creighton Calm in Face of Life Trial," *New York Evening Journal,* October 12, 1935; "Dr. Gettler on Stand at Appelgate Trial," *New York Times,* January 18, 1936, p. 6; "Mrs. Creighton Dies for Poison Murder: Appelgate Follows Her to the Death Chamber for the Slaying of His Wife," *New York Times,* July 17, 1936, p. 1.

**a picture of the two colleagues, taken about a year . . . :** Photographs provided by the family of Alexander O. Gettler.

## Epilogue: The Surest Poison

**"If any one person deserves . . .":** A. W. Freireich, "In Memoriam: Alexander O. Gettler 1883–1968," *Journal of Forensic Sciences* 14, no. 3 (July 1969), p. vii.

**what toxicologists now call "wet" chemistry . . . :** Henry C. Freimuth, "Alexander O. Gettler (1883–1968)," *American Journal of Forensic Medicine and Pathology* 4, no. 4 (December 1983).

**The work was so often grisly . . . :** Irving Sunshine, *Was It a Poisoning? Forensic Toxicologists Searching for Answers* (New York: American Academy of Forensic Scientists/Society of Forensic Toxicologists, 1998).

**"If they did not" . . . :** Ibid.

**"His interest in his former students . . .":** Freireich, "In Memoriam."

**His son, Joseph . . . :** Eugene Pawley, "Cause of Death: Ask Gettler," *American Mercury,* September 1954, pp. 62–66.

The employees of Thorndike Press hope you have enjoyed this Large Print book. All our Thorndike, Wheeler, and Kennebec Large Print titles are designed for easy reading, and all our books are made to last. Other Thorndike Press Large Print books are available at your library, through selected bookstores, or directly from us.

For information about titles, please call:
(800) 223-1244

or visit our Web site at:
http://gale.cengage.com/thorndike

To share your comments, please write:
Publisher
Thorndike Press
295 Kennedy Memorial Drive
Waterville, ME 04901